Navigating the
Complexities of Stroke

Lisa M. Shulman, MD
Editor-in-Chief, *Neurology Now*™ Book Series
Fellow of the American Academy of Neurology
Professor of Neurology
University of Maryland School of Medicine
Baltimore, MD

Other Titles in the *Neurology Now*™ Book Series

Navigating Life with Parkinson Disease
Sotirios A. Parashos, MD, PhD; Rose Wichmann, PT; and Todd Melby

Navigating Life with a Brain Tumor
Lynne P. Taylor, MD, FAAN; Alyx Porter Umphrey, MD; and Diane Richard

Navigating the Complexities of Stroke

Louis R. Caplan, MD

Professor of Neurology

Harvard University

Senior Neurologist

Beth Israel Deaconess Medical Center

Boston, MA

OXFORD

UNIVERSITY PRESS

OXFORD
UNIVERSITY PRESS

Oxford University Press is a department of the University of Oxford.
It furthers the University's objective of excellence in research, scholarship,
and education by publishing worldwide.

Oxford   New York
Auckland   Cape Town   Dar es Salaam   Hong Kong   Karachi
Kuala Lumpur   Madrid   Melbourne   Mexico City   Nairobi
New Delhi   Shanghai   Taipei   Toronto

With offices in
Argentina   Austria   Brazil   Chile   Czech Republic   France   Greece
Guatemala   Hungary   Italy   Japan   Poland   Portugal   Singapore
South Korea   Switzerland   Thailand   Turkey   Ukraine   Vietnam

Oxford is a registered trademark of Oxford University Press in the UK
and certain other countries.

Published in the United States of America by
Oxford University Press
198 Madison Avenue, New York, NY 10016

© American Academy of Neurology 2013

First issued as an Oxford University Press paperback, 2013

Library of Congress Cataloging-in-Publication Data
Caplan, Louis R.
Navigating the complexities of stroke / Louis R. Caplan, MD, professor of neurology,
Beth Israel Deaconess Medical Center, Boston, Massachusetts.
pages cm
Includes bibliographical references and index.
ISBN 978–0–19–994571–9 (alk. paper)
1. Cerebrovascular disease.   I. Title.
RC388.5.C3294 2014
616.8′1—dc23   2012043697

This material is not intended to be, and should not be considered, a substitute for medical or other professional
advice. Treatment for the conditions described in this material is highly dependent on the individual
circumstances. And, while this material is designed to offer accurate information with respect to the subject
matter covered and to be current as of the time it was written, research and knowledge about medical and health
issues is constantly evolving and dose schedules for medications are being revised continually, with new side
effects recognized and accounted for regularly. Readers must therefore always check the product information
and clinical procedures with the most up-to-date published product information and data sheets provided by
the manufacturers and the most recent codes of conduct and safety regulation. The publisher and the authors
make no representations or warranties to readers, express or implied, as to the accuracy or completeness of this
material. Without limiting the foregoing, the publisher and the authors make no representations or warranties
as to the accuracy or efficacy of the drug dosages mentioned in the material. The authors and the publisher do
not accept, and expressly disclaim, any responsibility for any liability, loss or risk that may be claimed or incurred
as a consequence of the use and/or application of any of the contents of this material.

Disclosure statements for potential conflicts of interest provided by the authors are available
upon request from the American Academy of Neurology, 201 Chicago Avenue, Minneapolis,
MN 55415; Attn: *Neurology Now Books*.

1 3 5 7 9 8 6 4 2
Printed in the United States of America
on acid-free paper

CONTENTS

ABOUT THE AAN'S *NEUROLOGY NOW*™ BOOK SERIES

Here is a question for you:

If you know more about your neurologic condition, will you do better than if you know less?

Well, not simply optimism but hard data show that individuals who are more knowledgeable about their medical conditions *do have better outcomes*. So learning about your neurologic condition plays an important role in doing the very best you can. The main purpose of both the American Academy of Neurology's (AAN's) *Neurology Now*™ book series and *Neurology Now* magazine is to focus on the needs of people with neurologic disorders. Our goal is to view neurologic issues through the eyes of people with neurologic problems, in order to understand and respond to their practical day-to-day needs.

So, you are probably saying, *"Of course, knowledge is a good thing, but how can it change the course of my disease?"* Well, health care is really a two-way street. You need to find a knowledgeable and trusted neurologist; however, no physician can overcome the obstacle of working with inaccurate or incomplete information. Your physician is working to navigate the clues you provide in your own words combined with the clues from their neurologic examination, in order to arrive at an accurate diagnosis and respond to your individual needs. Many types of important clues exist, such as your description of your symptoms or your ability to identify how your neurologic condition affects your daily activities. Poor patient–physician communication inevitably results in less-than-ideal outcomes. This problem is well described by the old adage, "garbage in, garbage out." The better you pin down and communicate your main problem(s), the more likely you are to walk out of your doctor's office with the plan that is right for you. Your neurologist is the expert in your disorder, but you and your family are the experts in "you." Physician decision making is not a "one shoe fits all" enterprise, yet when accurate, individualized information is lacking, that's what it becomes.

Whether you are startled by hearing a new diagnosis or you come to this knowledge gradually, learning that you have a neurologic problem is jarring. Many neurologic disorders are chronic; you aren't simply adjusting to something new—you will need to deal with this disorder for the foreseeable future. In certain ways, life has changed. Now, there are two crucial "next steps": the first is finding good neurologic care for your problem, and the second is successfully adjusting to living with your condition. This second step depends on attaining knowledge of your condition, learning new skills to manage the condition, and finding the flexibility and resourcefulness to restore your quality of life. When successful, you regain your equilibrium and restore a sense of confidence and control that is the cornerstone of well-being.

When healthy adjustment does not occur following a new diagnosis, a sense of feeling out of control and overwhelmed often persists, and no doctor's prescription will adequately respond to this problem. Individuals who acquire good self-management skills are often able to recognize and understand new symptoms and take appropriate action. Conversely, those who are lacking in confidence may respond to the same symptom with a growing sense of anxiety and urgency. In the first case, "watchful waiting" or a call to the physician may result in resolution of the problem. In the second case, the uncertainty and anxiety often lead to multiple physician consultations, unnecessary new prescriptions, social withdrawal, or unwarranted hospitalization. Outcomes can be dramatically different depending on knowledge and preparedness.

Managing a neurologic disorder is new territory, and you should not be surprised that you need to be equipped with new information and a new skill set to effectively manage your condition. You will need to learn new words that describe both your symptoms and their treatment to communicate effectively with the members of your medical team. You will also need to learn how to gather accurate information about your condition when you need it and to avoid misinformation. Although all of your physicians document your progress in their medical records, keeping a personal journal about your neurologic condition will help you summarize and track all your medical information in one place. When you bring this journal with you as you go to see your physician, you will be able to provide more accurate information about your history and previous treatment. Your active and informed involvement in your care and decision making results in a better quality of care and better outcomes.

Your neurologic condition is likely to pose new challenges in daily activities, including interactions in your family, your workplace, and your social and recreational activities. How can you best manage your symptoms or your medication dosing schedule in the context of your normal activities? When should you disclose your diagnosis to others? *Neurology Now* Books provide you with the background you need, including the experiences of others who have faced similar problems, to guide you through this unfamiliar terrain. Our goal is to give you the resources you need to "take your doctor with you" when you confront these new challenges. We are committed to answering the questions and concerns of individuals living with neurologic disorders and their families in each volume of the *Neurology Now* book series. We want you to be as prepared and confident as possible to participate with your doctors in your medical care. Much care is taken to develop each book with you in mind. We include the most up-to-date, informative, and useful answers to the questions that most concern you—whether you find yourself in the unexpected role of patient or caregiver. Real-life experiences of patients and families are found throughout the text to illustrate important points. And feedback based on correspondence from *Neurology Now* magazine readers informs topics for new books and is integral to our quality improvement. These features are found in all books in the *Neurology Now* book series so that you can expect the same quality and patient-centered approach in every volume.

I hope that you have arrived at a new understanding of why "knowledge is empowering" when it comes to your medical care and that *Neurology Now* Books will serve as an important foundation for the new skills you need to be effective in managing a neurologic condition.

Lisa M. Shulman, MD
Editor-in-Chief, *Neurology Now*™ Book Series
Fellow of the American Academy of Neurology
and Professor of Neurology
University of Maryland School of Medicine

FOREWORD

I'm not going sugar-coat this: strokes are awful. There's no getting around that fact. If you, like me, have had a stroke, you will agree. If you have a loved one who has had a stroke, you will also agree. I am telling you this not because I want to depress you, but because I want to be brutally honest. When I was 26, I lost speech, vision, the ability to walk, and the use of my hand. I got better, but it took many years. My stroke has shaken my family and friends. Recovery has been the biggest challenge of my life.

For stroke victims and their families, recovery is possible, but it can be very slow and the pace can be disheartening. So you have to become more patient than you were before. In my case, I had to do those blasted exercises again and again for hours a day, while all my friends were off in society becoming doctors and tycoons, getting married, and having kids.

The only way I was able to tolerate the trial of this stroke was that I had a really encouraging network of friends and family. When I encountered people who were not kind or encouraging, I departed. When a physical therapist told me, unasked, that I might never get rid of an ankle brace, I switched therapists. (I also got rid of my ankle brace.) I encourage patients to shop around if you are not satisfied with your care. Neuro rehab is very different from one city or hospital to another.

I found it helpful to compare my progress to the month before. Can my arm reach higher than this time last month? Do my words come out from the cobwebs of my mind more quickly? Am I still rude to waiters? (For a while after my stroke I lost my manners; now I am a pleasant dinner companion again.)

Reading about your stroke can be very helpful. I've found that learning about it from a height, as a detached student, makes it more manageable. I am also a patient of Dr. Caplan's. *Navigating the Complexities of Stroke* is designed to provide you with detailed guidance about the brain, the different kinds of strokes, their treatment, and the aftermath for patients and their caregivers. Having this information in one place can be very useful as you navigate rehabilitation and the medical bureaucracy. Anyone who is at risk of stroke, those who care for stroke patients, and patients themselves can all gain wisdom from this book.

When I see Dr. Caplan, he usually tells me to get on with my life. In that vein, I encourage you not to think about your stroke all the time. This is hard because so much of your brain and body is broken. Try to have adventures and fun. Surround yourself with people who love you, even if you are less nimble than before.

Nina Mitchell
Boston, MA
(Nina's stroke website is at http://mindpop.net.)

PREFACE

This is the second edition of a monograph commissioned by the American Academy of Neurology that aims to inform the public about stroke. Recognizing that readers will have diverse educational backgrounds and medical experience, I have tried to make the book useful for all levels of readers. Stroke is complex. The organ involved, the brain, is the most diverse and complex of all of the body's structures. I have tried in this book to capture that complexity and still render enough easily digested information to make it useful for all readers.

As in the first edition, I use individual patients to illustrate different types of stroke. After introducing four patients, I add information about their symptoms, evaluation, and treatment in the chapters devoted to those topics. I then summarize their cases at the end of the book. Individual cases help readers understand the general principles discussed.

I believe this edition represents a major upgrade from the previous publication. I have added a chapter on strokes in babies, children, and young adults. I have added new information and illustrations in each of the other chapters. I have completely reordered the chapters. The brain and its functions and blood supply are now placed first, after the Introduction. One of the major reasons that the public in general is less knowledgeable about stroke compared to cancer and heart disease is the complexity of the brain and the diversity of symptoms. By discussing the brain and its anatomy and functions first, I aim to clarify why certain symptoms occur and what they mean.

Publication of printed materials has also changed dramatically since the first edition in 2006. Oxford University Press, one of the world leaders in medical publications for doctors and the public, will make this material widely available as an e-book and for iPads and other devices.

I hope in some small way the information in this book helps readers prevent strokes and arms them and their families to navigate the complexities of their medical care and recovery.

Louis R. Caplan, MD
Boston, MA
Fall 2012

Navigating the Complexities of Stroke

Chapter 1

Introduction

Why Is Stroke So Important?

"It was then that it happened. To my shock and incredulity, I could not speak. That is, I could utter nothing intelligible. All that would come from my lips was the sound *ab* which I repeated again and again...Then as I watched it, the telephone handpiece slid slowly from my grasp, and I, in turn, slid slowly from my chair and landed on the floor behind the desk...At 5:15 in that January dusk I had been a person; now at 6:45 I was a case. But I found it easy to accept my altered condition. I felt like a case."

—ERIC HODGINS *(Hodgins E.* Episode: Report on the Accident Inside My Skull. *New York: Atheneum; 1964:7–14.)*

Effect of Strokes on Individuals

When speakers and writers stress the importance of stroke, they usually quote numbers and statistics. But to me the most important aspect of stroke is its effect on the individual person who develops a stroke. What is more frightening and devastating than to suddenly become unable to speak, understand speech, move an arm or leg, stand, walk, balance, hear, see, read, feel, write, or remember? Loss of function is often instantaneous and totally unanticipated. The first common term for stroke, **apoplexy**, literally meant "struck suddenly with violence" in Greek. The word **stroke** refers to being suddenly stricken. Losing brain function can be dehumanizing and often makes individuals dependent on others for ordinary daily activities. The brain is without question the most important organ in the human body. It is responsible for our movements, feelings, moods, thoughts, and perceptions, and it enables our unique personal characteristics, our abilities and failings, our intelligence, our feelings, and our personalities. Our brains make us what we are. The loss of any brain function diminishes the person in us. In surveys that ask individuals about their worst health fears, most people rate cancer and stroke at the top of their lists. People worry about the pain of cancer and fear losing their mental and physical functions and becoming dependent on others if they were to have a stroke. Everyone would like to exit this life with their capabilities and mind intact, despite the inevitable aging of their bodies.

The quote at the beginning of this chapter was written by a famous writer, Eric Hodgins, the author of a once very popular best seller, *Mr. Blandings Builds His Dream House*. In Hodgins's later book, *Episode: Report on the Accident inside My Skull*, he describes exactly what it felt like to be suddenly deprived of speech and movement of his right limbs. He changed from a highly functioning human being in one moment to a helpless, dumb invalid—"a case"—in the next instant. Imagine an articulate author dependent for his livelihood on his use of language, becoming totally unable to speak or write.

The Complexity of Stroke

Stroke is a complicated condition. Strokes have many different causes and have very different effects on individuals. Loss of function may be temporary or permanent, slight or devastating. Some functions may improve while others remain impaired. It will prove easier for readers to understand explanations about stroke if they are able to follow individuals who have had strokes. For that reason, I now introduce four stroke patients. I will refer throughout the book to these individuals: their symptoms, stroke risk factors, the causes of their strokes, their evaluations and treatments, and the effects that their strokes had on themselves and their families and environment.

Robert H., a 68-year-old retired engineer, lived with his wife. His three children were married and no longer lived at home. He had had many health problems during the past. His blood pressure was discovered to be high 20 years ago. He had been given a number of different pills, but high blood pressure remained a problem that was not always well controlled. Ten years ago he had a heart attack and had to have surgery on his coronary arteries. For the past few years he has felt pain in the right calf of his leg when he walks. His doctors told him that an artery to that leg had narrowed. Similar blood pressure and heart problems had led to his father dying at age 51. His brother also had hypertension and had had several heart attacks. One sister had had a stroke.

One day at work, Robert noticed that his left hand and arm felt numb and that he could not hold objects in that hand. The weakness and numbness lasted about 15 minutes. He assumed that he had leaned on that hand. Two days later, shortly after he awakened in the morning, his left face and hand felt numb and tingly for about 5 minutes. That afternoon, a shade seemed to come over his right eye, and he could not see from that eye for about a minute. These symptoms worried him and he scheduled appointments with his eye doctor and primary physician. Two days later, before he saw either doctor, when he tried to get out of bed in the morning he fell on the floor. His wife heard the fall and rushed to him. She recognized that his left limbs could not move, but Robert seemed unaware of the nature of the problem. She called an ambulance and rushed him to the emergency room of the hospital.

Claire H., a 29-year-old lawyer, began to notice intermittent pain in her left face and neck. The pain was often sharp and was sometimes accompanied by headache. She lived at home with her husband and two small children. She was very athletic and played ice hockey on a team several nights a week. Her health had been excellent. She took no medications and a recent checkup showed no health problems. One of her uncles has had lung cancer, but there was no history of heart disease or stroke in her parents, their siblings, or her own three brothers, all of whom were older than her.

Three days after the onset of the neck and face pain, Claire began to hear a pulsing sound in her left ear. Later that day, her right hand and arm went weak and she could not speak well. Her husband collected her at work and drove her to the hospital.

Tom M., a 61-year-old single man, became ill at work. He was a longshoreman who did heavy physical work. While straining to lift some heavy cargo, he felt dizzy and lurched to his left. He staggered and seemed "drunk" to his coworkers. Several minutes later he vomited and reported that he had developed a bad headache in the back of his head and pain in his left neck and shoulder.

In the past he had been healthy but he admitted to drinking wine rather heavily. He did not visit doctors regularly. When checked by the company doctor 4 years previously, Tom was told that his blood pressure was "a bit high" and would need to be rechecked, but he had not followed through.

Elaine S. was an 82-year-old woman. Her health had always been good. She was a widow who lived a very active life and often babysat for her grandchildren. Recently she noticed episodes in which her heart beat fast and irregularly. This would last from 2 to 15 minutes and worried her, but she did not tell her doctor. One afternoon her left hand and leg suddenly went weak, and she felt tingling over the entire left side of her body, including her face. She immediately went to the hospital.

I will have much more to say about these individuals in the various chapters in this book. In Chapter 16, I will summarize their cases.

Numbers

Stroke is and has been the third leading cause of death in most countries for a very long time. Only heart disease and cancer are bigger killers. Strokes are a more important cause of prolonged disability than any other medical condition. Survivors of strokes are often unable to return to work or to assume their former effectiveness as spouses, parents, friends, and active participants in their communities.

In the United States, nearly 800,000 individuals have a stroke, and 150,000 (90,000 women and 60,000 men) die from stroke, each year. Three-fourths of the strokes each year are first strokes and one-fourth are recurrent strokes (Heart disease and stroke statistics—2010 update. A report from the American Heart Association. Circulation. 2010;121:e46–e215). At any one time, there are about two million stroke survivors living in the United States. In China, approximately 2.5 million people have a stroke each year, and 1.5 million people die each year because of stroke. Someone in the United States has a stroke every 40 seconds, and every 4 minutes someone dies of stroke. Every year about 55,000 more women than men have a stroke. Stroke affects three times as many women as breast cancer and yet receives much less public attention. Stroke is the second most common cause of death in the world surpassed as a killer only by heart disease. Strokes are an even more important cause of prolonged disability. A stroke often renders individuals unable to return to work or to assume their former effectiveness as spouses, parents, friends, and citizens. The economic, social, and psychological costs of stroke are enormous. The estimated cost of stroke in the United States in 2010 was $73.7 billion.

Many people think that strokes only happen to old folks, but they occur at all ages including infancy, childhood, adolescence, and early adulthood. One of the patients mentioned so far, Claire, was only 29 when she had her stroke. During the last 40 years I have taken care of over 200 patients who have had strokes before their fortieth birthday. Although it is true that strokes are much more common in people over 65, they also often occur in younger individuals. There are now several medical books devoted entirely to discussions of strokes in children and young people. Stroke can happen to anyone. Stroke can happen to you!

Strokes in History

The history of the world has undoubtedly been greatly affected and altered by stroke. Many important leaders in science, art, medicine, and politics have had their productivity cut prematurely short by stroke. Louis Pasteur, the great French scientist whose discoveries led to vaccinations to prevent smallpox, had a stroke at age 46 that caused left-sided paralysis, although he continued to make important advances until additional strokes impaired his function at age 65. Marcello Malpighi, one of the first individuals to describe the biological characteristics of small blood vessels and capillaries and to write about the anatomy of the lungs, kidneys, and spleen as seen under a microscope, died of a stroke that had paralyzed his right arm and leg.

Two very important political leaders during the early twentieth century, Vladimir Lenin and Woodrow Wilson, had intellectual impairments related to stroke while they were at the helms of their countries at critical times in history. At age 52, Lenin had a sudden onset of slurred speech and right-sided paralysis. An observer noted that as he spoke, the words were often slurred, and he paused several times like a man who has lost the thread of his argument. When he died, his brain showed multiple strokes and his blood vessels were described as being hard as stone. Woodrow Wilson, president of the United States and the architect of the League of Nations during the first quarter of the twentieth century, had a series of small strokes that left him with difficulty speaking and swallowing and with left arm and leg weakness at a time when he was working hard for world peace and cooperation. All of the heads of state who met at Yalta and elsewhere to divide up the spheres of influence after World War II—Franklin Roosevelt (United States), Winston Churchill (Great Britain), and Josef Stalin (Russia)—had

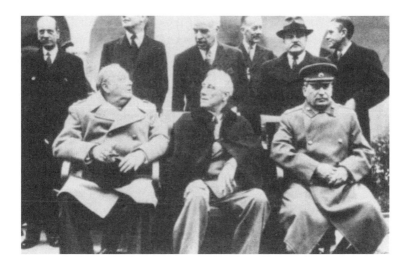

FIGURE 1-1 Roosevelt, Churchill, and Stalin at Yalta. The three leaders of their respective countries all had advanced cerebrovascular disease.

severe **cerebrovascular disease** at the time of their meetings and would have multiple strokes. Figure 1-1 is a photograph that shows these three leaders at a conference. Roosevelt subsequently died of a fatal stroke due to brain hemorrhage after years of very severe hypertension. In Roosevelt's time there was no very effective treatment for high blood pressure. History might have been very different if the brains of these leaders had not been addled by stroke. Public awareness of stroke increased dramatically when President Dwight Eisenhower developed a stroke that caused his speech to slur and when President Richard Nixon died after a large acute stroke.

The Plan of This Stroke Primer

I began this book by emphasizing the importance of stroke in this introductory chapter, both in general and for individuals. The next two chapters form the foundation of information needed to understand the main findings in stroke patients: what the brain looks like and how it works, and the blood vessels that supply the brain. The five chapters following these describe the different kinds of stroke, their causes, stroke and cerebrovascular conditions in the young, symptoms and findings in stroke patients, and risk factors for stroke. The remaining chapters are about the evaluation of stroke patients and methods of treating and preventing strokes.

Chapter 2

What Does the Brain Look Like and How Does It Work?

"From the brain, and from the brain only, arise our pleasures, joys, laughter, and jests, as well as our sorrows, pains, griefs and tears."

—HIPPOCRATES

The brain is the organ that malfunctions in stroke patients. Knowledge about the brain, and how it looks and acts, can help individuals understand stroke symptoms, abnormalities, and handicaps. This chapter introduces readers to brain anatomy and function. The vocabulary that doctors use to explain things to stroke patients and their families often contains anatomical and functional terms. I hope that this chapter will make it easier for readers to follow the explanations that doctors and other health care professionals offer.

The brain is without question the most important and yet also the most complicated human organ. The brain controls movements, feelings, moods, thoughts, and perceptions. The brain makes it possible to explore the environment and to interact with others. Seeing, hearing, touching, speaking, and communicating are all brain functions. The brain is what makes our characters, our abilities and failings, our intelligence, our feelings, and our personalities. Our brains make us what we are.

The brain is the most intricate and complex computer yet known. I will explore the brain with the readers first by describing and illustrating what it looks like from the outside, and then by describing the inside of the brain and its various parts. While discussing and illustrating its anatomy, I will describe as simply as possible what is known about the functions of the various parts of the brain.

The Appearance of the Brain

External Surface

The Cerebral Hemispheres

Figure 2-1 is a side view of the brain from the left side. Figure 2.2 shows the outside of the brain from the top. The largest part of the brain shown in these figures is called the **cerebrum.** The largest portion of the brain overall, it consists of two halves. The two sides of the cerebrum are called the left and right **cerebral hemispheres.** The hemispheres are separated into divisions called lobes. The different lobes of the cerebral hemispheres are shaded differently on

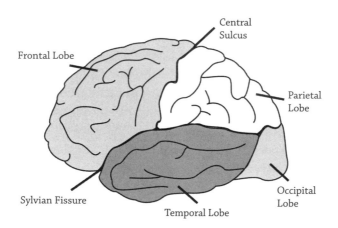

FIGURE 2-1 Side view of the cerebrum from the left side.

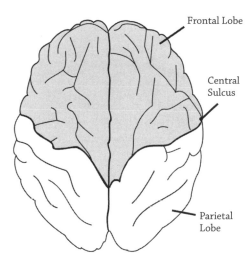

FIGURE 2-2 View of the cerebral hemispheres from the top.

the illustrations to help identify them. These figures show just the surface of the cerebral hemispheres, not the deeper parts inside. They do not show the **brainstem** (the portion of the brain that connects the cerebrum to the spinal cord) or the **cerebellum** (literally the "little brain," the portion of the brain located in the back of the head that is attached to the brainstem). The latter two structures are further back and below the cerebrum, which covers them much like the cap of a mushroom hovers over the rest of it. A side view of the brain with the brainstem and cerebellum and spinal cord attached is shown in Figure 2-3.

The surface of the cerebral and cerebellar hemispheres is made up of folded, raised strips of brain tissue called gyri. Between the gyri are valleys or clefts called sulci. A black line is drawn on Figure 2-1 along the central sulcus. The frontal lobe lies in front of the central sulcus, and the parietal lobe, temporal lobe, and occipital lobe lie behind the central sulcus. These names are derived from common terms for the bony parts of the head: *frontal* from the front of the head behind the forehead; the *temporal* lobes lie behind

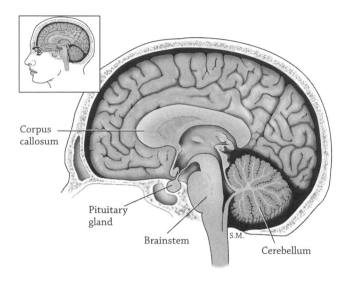

FIGURE 2-3 View of the paramedial portion of the left cerebral hemisphere, and the brainstem, cerebellum, and upper spinal cord.

the temples; the term *parietal* means "outside" or "away from the center," and *occipital* comes from the Latin words for "back of the head": *occi caput.*

The Brainstem

Figure 2-3 is a left-side view that shows the location of the brainstem and cerebellum in relation to the left cerebral hemisphere. Figure 2-4 is a view of the underside of the brain that shows the position of the brainstem and its connection with the spinal cord. Cross sections of the different parts of the brainstem are illustrated in Figure 2-5. The brainstem is a relatively small but very critical structure located in the back of the head under the cerebrum; it connects the spinal cord below with the cerebrum above as an upward continuation of the spinal cord. The lowest, most caudal (toward

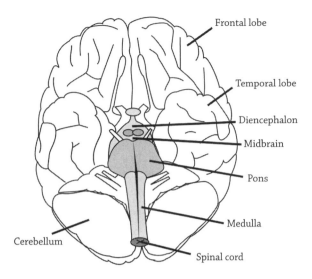

Frontal lobe

Temporal lobe

Diencephalon

Midbrain

Pons

Medulla

Cerebellum

Spinal cord

FIGURE 2-4 View of the undersurface of the brain.

the tail) portion of the brainstem is called the **medulla oblongata.** This connects to the **pons,** named after the Latin word for bridge because of its appearance. The most rostral (toward the front of the head) portion of the brainstem is called the **midbrain** or mesencephalon. Above the midbrain is the **thalamus,** a region also referred to as the diencephalon. The brainstem has five major functions: (1) it contains nerve cells and nerves that relate to the head and face and their movements and senses; (2) it acts as a pathway for information traveling to and from the cerebral hemispheres; (3) it acts as a relay station for information coming to and from the cerebellum; (4) it contains nerve cells and pathways that maintain consciousness and alertness and relate to sleep and wakefulness; and (5) it houses nerve cells, located in the lower brainstem, that control automatic body functions such as breathing, heart rate, and blood pressure. Destruction of the brainstem leads to loss of all brain functions, coma, and death.

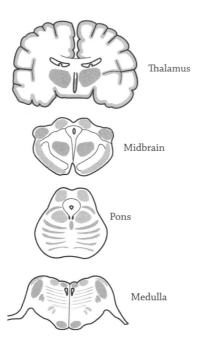

Thalamus

Midbrain

Pons

Medulla

FIGURE 2-5 Cross sections through the parts of the brainstem: thalamus, midbrain, pons, medulla.

The Cerebellum

The cerebellum, whose name literally means "little cerebrum" or "little brain," looks like a small walnut that is attached to the brainstem and is placed far back in the head, below and behind the cerebrum, which dwarfs the cerebellum in size. The cerebellum helps coordinate all body movements—those of the limbs, eyes, and mouth.

Internal Appearance and Composition

Figure 2-6 shows a cut section of the brain. The cerebral cortex is the gray ribbon on the very periphery of the section. Many of the nerve cells that relate to the brain's various motor, sensory, cognitive, and

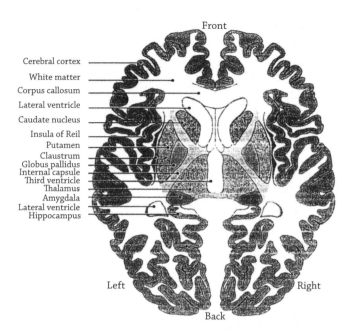

Front

Cerebral cortex
White matter
Corpus callosum
Lateral ventricle
Caudate nucleus
Insula of Reil
Putamen
Claustrum
Globus pallidus
Internal capsule
Third ventricle
Thalamus
Amygdala
Lateral ventricle
Hippocampus

Left   Right

Back

FIGURE 2-6 A cut section through the cerebrum.

behavioral functions are located in the cerebral cortex. These cortical nerve cells (called neurons) give rise to nerve fibers that communicate with other cerebral cortical regions. Fibers also travel from these cortical neurons downward toward the gray nuclei imbedded within the brain (often called basal ganglia), and also to neurons located in the brainstem, cerebellum, and spinal cord. The basal ganglia are composed of three separate but closely interrelated structures: the caudate nucleus, globus pallidus, and putamen. The caudate nucleus and putamen are often linked together as the lentiform nucleus.

Many nerve fibers travel upward from the spinal cord, brainstem, cerebellum, and basal ganglia toward the cerebral cortex, mostly to relay information about the external environment and the body's internal environment. The fibers are covered with a fatty enveloping substance called myelin, which imparts a white color to the region under the cerebral cortex that gives rise to the term *white matter*. The myelin allows faster transmission of nerve impulses through the nerve fibers, much like insulation around an ordinary electric wire facilitates transmission of electrical energy. Fibers travelling away from neurons are called axons and are characterized as **efferent,** meaning that they travel centrifugally, while fibers travelling toward the neurons are called dendrites and are referred to as **afferent** because they travel centripetally.

Afferent and efferent fibers are organized into bundles called tracts that resemble roads leading into and out of the various groups of neurons. When fibers connect with other nerve cells they transmit their message by way of a variety of special chemicals called neurotransmitters in a communication region called a synapse. Neurons and their fibers are shown in Figure 2-7.

The brainstem can be compared to a small village that lies outside a major urban city, a kind of bedroom community. Major highways going into and out of the city must travel through this village. These roads are situated on the outside of the village to facilitate travel. Similarly, the long motor tracts leading from the cerebrum (e.g., the major motor pathways located in the internal capsule shown in Figure 2-6) travel in the base of the brainstem through areas named after their locale (e.g., the cerebral peduncle, basis pontis, and medullary pyramid) and continue as the pyramidal tracts in the spinal cord. The main sensory tracts also travel in peripheral zones of the brainstem on their way to the thalamus.

The village also has local shops and local traffic of its own. The village can be thought of as the head with all of its organs, movements, and attached special senses. Businesses (groups of nerve cells and nuclei) are located mostly in the dorsal portion of the brainstem called the tegmentum. Some brainstem motor nuclei control eye, tongue, face, and neck movements, while others receive sensory input related to sounds; movement in space; and touch, pain, temperature, and pressure felt in the face, throat, mouth, nose, ears, and so forth. These things all relate to local business in the village (the head organs).

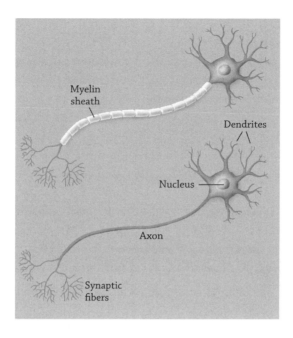

FIGURE 2-7 Nerve cells, axons, and myelin.

The cerebellum can be thought of as a separate structure (perhaps a specialized health club) that is located outside of the village. It can only be reached through the village by three different roads (the superior, middle, and inferior cerebellar peduncles), which attach to the brainstem in its lower (medulla), middle (pons), and upper (midbrain) portions. The cerebellum aids coordination of various eye, neck, tongue, and body movements. The cerebellum intimately relates to the **vestibular** system in the brainstem. The peripheral receptors for the vestibular system are located within the inner ear. They relate to a series of canals shaped like tires. Movement of the head and neck shifts the fluid in these canals and tells the individual precise information about the relation of their head to space. This type of information about motion and localization in space is absolutely critical for birds and fish. Humans get this type of information from a number of inputs, including the vestibular system, vision, and joint position sense. Information goes from the inner ears in the vestibular nerves to the vestibular nuclei located within the brainstem tegmentum. This information then goes to the nuclei that control eye movements so that your eyes move along with your head, allowing you to continue to focus while running, swimming, or turning. It also goes to the cerebellum to help coordinate walking and use of the limbs. The cerebellum sends information to the cerebrum and to the spinal cord nerve cells by way of the brainstem.

Alertness is maintained by a series of small neurons located on each side near the middle of the brainstem tegmentum called the reticular activating system. These nerve cells send messages through the thalamus to each side of the cerebrum to maintain alertness and an awake, energized state. If the reticular activating system on both sides of the brainstem is injured, then coma develops. This system, along with other nuclei located in the upper brainstem, also controls the sleep-wake cycle.

Brain Functions

Most organs, like the liver, lungs, and skin, are relatively homogeneous. One part of these organs looks and works the same as another. Not so in the brain. Structures and functions in the brain are quite well localized. The various brain regions look different, function differently, and contain different chemical substances called neurotransmitters that are used to transfer information from one nerve cell to another. For instance, moving a limb, feeling a coin in a hand, seeing, talking, reading, smelling, walking, and hearing, to mention only some key body activities, are all localized to very different but characteristic brain regions. To make things even more complex, the sides of the body, and even the functions of the individual limbs—the shoulder, arm, hand, thigh, leg, and foot—have different localizations within the brain.

The left side of the brain generally controls activities of the right arm and leg and is involved in perception and analysis of various stimuli (feeling, sound, visual objects) that are presented to the right side of the body and the right side of space outside of the body. The right side of the brain controls the same functions on the left side of the body. Many psychological and general medical problems give general symptoms of brain dysfunction, such as feeling low, tired, sleepy, confused, generally weak, and so forth. The most common disorder affecting a local region of the brain is stroke.

Motor Functions (Movement, Strength, Coordination, Walking)

In general, the parts of the brain in front of the central sulcus (the frontal lobes) are mostly related to action and movement, so-called **motor** functions, while the area behind the central sulcus are more involved with sensory input. Figure 2-8 shows the location of the motor and sensory cerebral cortex on each side of the central sulcus (B) and the efferent motor pathway that originates from the primary motor cortex (A). The efferent pathway from the motor cortex neurons is called the cortico-spinal or pyramidal tract. This tract descends within the white matter under the cortex (called the centrum semi-ovale) into the white matter near the deep gray nuclei (called the corona radiata). The tract then courses through the front portion of the internal capsule, a white matter tract that lies like a road with a single, nearly 45-degree bend between various basal gray nuclei. The tract then descends within the basal portion of the brainstem; fibers within the pyramidal tract will leave the main path to synapse with the various nuclei within the brainstem that innervate movements of the eyes, face, jaw, and tongue. The pyramidal tract then descends into the spinal cord to synapse with motor neurons within the anterior horns of the spinal cord that innervate the muscles of the trunk and limbs. Fibers that influence voluntary movement of the upper limbs will leave the tract in the upper neck

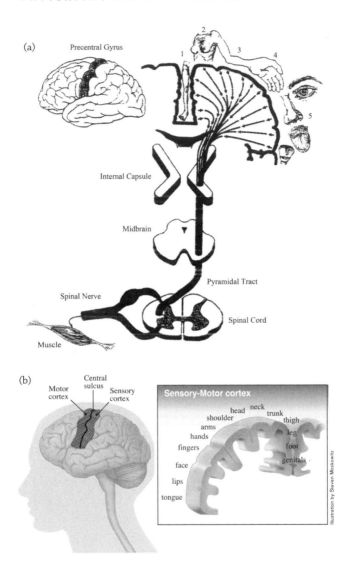

FIGURE 2-8   a: The motor system. b: The location of the motor cortex, central sulcus, and the sensory-motor cortex. The detailed insert shows the parts of the body represented along the motor cortex.

(cervical portion of the spinal cord) while fibers that influence the lower limbs leave the tract in the lower back (lumbar region). Some fibers within this descending motor tract go all the way to the lower end of the spinal cord (sacral or tail region) and synapse with nerve cells that help control the pelvic and genital muscles that relate to urination, defecation, and sexual function. Figure 2-9 shows the spinal cord and the location of the motor and sensory tracts within the spinal cord.

Damage to the motor cortex or the corticospinal (pyramidal) tract pathway at any point leads to loss of voluntary motor control of any parts located below the interruption. When individuals' pyramidal tract or the fibers leading into it are interrupted, they will not be able to move their arm, hand, and leg at will. The parts of the motor system are labeled directly on Figure 2-8. Patients Robert H., Claire H., and Elaine S. all had strokes that affected the motor systems of one of their cerebral hemispheres, leading to weakness on the side of the body opposite to their brain damage. In Chapter 9,

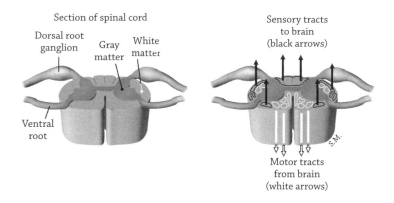

FIGURE 2-9 The anatomy of a cross section of the spinal cord, and the general location of the motor and sensory tracts in the spinal cord.

which discusses the evaluation of these patients, I will elaborate further on what their brain images showed and which portions of the motor system was involved in each patient.

The basal ganglia and the substantia nigra (a black nucleus in the midbrain whose loss of function contributes to Parkinson's disease) also influence motor functions. They are most concerned with automatic functions that individuals perform without having to think about doing them. Standing and sitting posture, position and movement of the arms and legs while walking, and facial expression are influenced greatly by basal ganglia nerve cells. The basal ganglia also has important functions in relation to whole-body movements such as sitting down, rising from a chair, and turning in bed. The cerebellum acts to coordinate and fine-tune movements and actions initiated through the basal ganglia and cortico-spinal systems. The coordination of eye movements, speech, movements of the arms and legs, and walking are influenced greatly by the cerebellum. Patient Tom M. staggered and lurched because his cerebellum was involved in his stroke.

Sensory Functions

The parts of the cerebrum behind the central sulcus (the parietal, temporal, and occipital lobes) are more related to **sensory** functions: perceptions of various stimuli in the environment such as vision, sound, and touch. In contrast to the predominantly efferent (i.e., outgoing) motor system are the sensory systems, which convey information to the cerebral cortex so that individuals can become consciously aware of what they see, hear, feel, taste, and smell. Other input tells them about movement within space and the relation of their body to space.

Sensory receptors on the periphery (within the eyes, ears, nose, tongue, and skin) first receive input from the environment. The information is sent to specific nuclei within the thalamus that are specialized for feeling, vision, hearing, motion, taste, and smell.

The information is then relayed to specialized regions within the cerebrum.

The **somatosensory** receptors within the skin, bones, and joints send information to neurons within nerve ganglia that lie outside the spinal cord. These neurons send information about touch, pain, heat, cold, pressure, and the location of the limbs in space toward the brain. They also send information locally to the motor nerve cells so that automatic reactions (reflexes) such as limb withdrawal can occur without the need for the information to pass through the brain. The tracts for pain and temperature sensation (spino-thalamic tracts) cross to the opposite side of the spinal cord and then ascend towards a very large, centrally located structure called the thalamus, which sits on top of the brainstem and at the foot of the cerebral hemispheres and is the main way station or relay for sensory input to the brain. Sensors specialized for motion and position of joints and limbs send information through a different pathway. The sensory ganglia send information in one of two tracts in the back portion of the spinal cord called the posterior columns. These fibers cross in the brainstem and form a tract called the medial lemniscus, which also travels to the sensory nuclei in the thalamus. Fibers from these two systems both synapse in nuclei in the lateral parts of the thalamus. The sensory information is then transmitted from the thalamic nuclei to a somatosensory area in the parietal lobe located in and around the postcentral gyrus. When the information reaches the brain, the individual becomes aware of sensory input and changes on the opposite side of their body. Figure 2-10 is a cartoon that shows the pathways for transmission of motor and sensory information to and from the left arm.

The visual and auditory systems have a similar pattern of relay of important information to the conscious brain. In each, information is first perceived in peripheral receptor nerve cells in the eye (retina) and inner ear (cochlea). Information then goes through the brain toward special nuclei in the thalamus, from where it is relayed to specialized regions in the brain. Regarding visual input

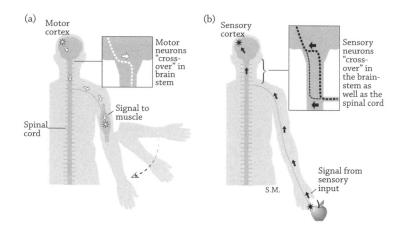

FIGURE 2-10   The pathways of the motor system (a) and sensory systems (b) in relation to movement and feeling in the left arm.

(Figure 2-11), the information from each eye travels through the optic nerve behind the eye. Fibers conveying information about visual stimuli that comes from the outer parts of vision (called temporal fields because they are closer to the temple) travel in the inner portions of each optic nerve, while fibers conveying visual data about the inner parts of the visual field (called nasal fields because they are closer to the nose) travel in the outer portions of each optic nerve. The inner fibers in each optic nerve then cross in an X-shaped structure near the pituitary gland called the optic chiasm. As you can see from Figure 2-11, this crossing realigns the visual fibers so that visual information related to the right side of vision in each eye is grouped in a fiber bundle that travels at the base of the left side of the brain called the optic tract. This tract contains information from the right temporal visual field and the left nasal field; that is, if you drew a line right in the middle of your vision, everything that is on the right would be contained in the left optic tract. Similarly, the right optic tract

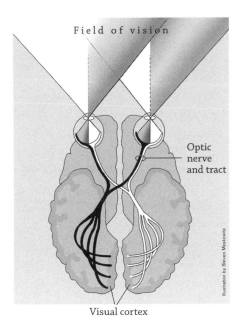

Field of vision

Optic nerve and tract

Visual cortex

FIGURE 2-11 The visual system pathways.

contains information from all the visual stimuli on your left (left temporal field and right nasal field). Each optic tract synapses in a specialized visual nucleus in the back and lateral portion of the thalamus on each side called the lateral geniculate bodies. In turn, fibers travel on each side within the back part of the brain in the visual radiations (called the geniculo-calcarine tracts) to end up in the visual cortex in the occipital lobe. The left visual cortex receives visual information from the right side of visual space and the right visual (striate) cortex receives information from left visual space. The concept that the brain is organized in relation to the sides of visual space is very hard for laypeople to grasp, since they tend to think of vision solely in relation to the individual eyes. As can be seen from the diagram, an abnormality in the right eye or right optic nerve will lead to loss of vision in that eye. In contrast, an abnormality in the right optic tract, lateral geniculate body, visual radiations, or visual cortex will lead to vision loss in the left side of visual space.

Sound input comes in through nerve cells in the inner ear and travels within the auditory nerves to nuclei located in the lateral portion of the brainstem (pons) on each side. These nuclei are appropriately named the auditory nuclei. Information is then relayed through a number of brainstem nuclei, finally arriving at specialized nuclei on each side of the thalamus called the medial geniculate bodies that lie near but inside of the specialized visual nuclei. From here the information is relayed to a specialized hearing cortex in each temporal lobe called Heschl's gyri, after the individual who discovered their functions. The right temporal lobe receives information from the left side of auditory space, while the left temporal lobe subserves right auditory space. Similar to the visual system, if an abnormality develops in a person's left ear or left auditory nerve then he or she will have difficulty hearing sounds exposed to the left ear, while an injury to his or her left medial geniculate body or left temporal lobe will involve all sound coming from the right side of auditory space, regardless of which ear hears the sounds.

There is a common pattern of specialization of each sensation within the cerebral cortex. Simple stimuli are received first in primary cortical regions that are named by the nature of the stimulus followed by a 1. For example, the primary visual cortex is called V_1, the primary auditory cortex is called A_1, and touch (somatosensory input) is first received at S_1. The stimuli that reach these primary areas are usually very simple. For example, V_1 receives stimuli of spots, lights, lines, and the like; A_1 receives simple sounds and noises, and S_1 receives simple touches and pressures on the skin.

Adjacent to these primary sensory regions are secondary sensory cortical regions in which more elaborate sensory information

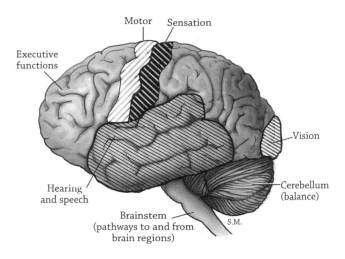

Motor Sensation
Executive functions
Vision
Hearing and speech
Cerebellum (balance)
Brainstem (pathways to and from brain regions)
S.M.

FIGURE 2-12 The location of some specialized brain regions.

is analyzed and processed. In the visual sphere, these might be boxes, circles, forms, and so forth. Adjacent to the secondary cortical regions are tertiary zones that process even more complex information: faces, animals, and scenes in the visual sphere, and words and musical phrases in the auditory sphere.

The various cortical zones described are labeled on Figure 2-12 The visual cortical zones are mostly located in the occipital lobes, the somatosensory cortical areas are located in the parietal lobes, and the auditory regions are located in the temporal lobes. Smell and taste are also localized to the temporal lobes.

The thalamus also connects to regions of the cerebral cortex on each side that have specialized abilities for memory, language, and visual-spatial and other cognitive and behavioral functions. The connections are organized as circuits in which there is reciprocal connectivity between the thalami, basal ganglia, substantia nigra, and different regions of the cerebral cortex.

Language and Speech

Language is extremely important for daily communication. The ability to use written language, to read, write, and spell, separates humans from all other species. I can vividly remember the great frustration that I felt when trying to obtain directions in Japan; the individuals I asked could not speak any English and I could not speak, understand, or read Japanese. We simply could not communicate with each other despite earnest effort on both sides. This experience is probably similar to what happens daily to patients who have severe loss of language abilities. **Aphasia** is the term used for loss of language capabilities. Speech consists of two different components: language, and mechanical movements of the mouth, lips, and tongue that allow individuals to articulate their language. Language functions are mostly localized to a region surrounding the large fissure that separates the frontal and temporal lobes on the outer surface of the brain (the sylvian fissure) in the so-called dominant hemisphere of the brain. The hemisphere that is dominant for speech is nearly always the left cerebral hemisphere in right-handed individuals and in 80 percent of left-handers. Individuals who are left handed are more likely to have some speech functions in each hemisphere. These latter individuals have aphasia when either hemisphere is involved, but the aphasia is less severe than if speech only resided on one side. Women more often have bilateral speech representation than men. The language zone is labeled in Figure 2-12.

Voluntary motor control of the face and limbs on the opposite side of the body is localized to the motor strip located in the precentral gyrus. The bottom of this region, just near the sylvian fissure below it, is specialized for voluntary control of the muscles of the face, tongue, cheeks, and pharynx. The so-called motor speech region, usually referred to as Broca's area, after French physician and anthropologist Paul Broca, is located just below and behind this motor region. This area is located in the third frontal gyrus in a triangular region that forms a lip over the sylvian fissure (the frontal operculum). Individuals who have injuries, infarcts, or hemorrhages in this general region, including the regions around Broca's area, often have difficulty producing normal speech. Their speech output is reduced and effortful and letters and words are poorly pronounced. The speech produced is usually accurate but not grammatically correct. Writing may also be agrammatical and telegraphic. This type of abnormality is usually referred to as Broca's aphasia. Most patients with this problem also have some degree of paralysis of their right hand, arm, and face.

Hearing is localized within the temporal lobes on each side. Next to this region in the dominant temporal lobe are cortical areas specialized for the understanding of spoken language. This region in the back portion of the superior temporal gyrus is usually called Wernicke's area after German neurologist Carl Wernicke, who was a pioneer in the study of language and the brain. Individuals with stroke-related damage to this region use wrong and sometimes nonexistent words and have difficulty repeating and understanding what is said to them. They may also not be able to understand what they read. Their writing also contains many wrong words. Damage limited to brain regions near Wernicke's area can cause the patient difficulty in repeating spoken language with relative preservation of understanding of speech (so-called conduction aphasia). Some individuals with very small lesions in the temporal lobe have a selective problem hearing words, even though they can hear and identify sounds well and can speak almost normally (pure word deafness). Others appear as if they are deaf to language and other sound input, although they jump and blink reflexively at loud, unexpected noises in their environment (cortical deafness).

Written language is mostly localized to a region surrounding the angular gyrus in the inferior back portion of the parietal lobe within the dominant cerebral hemisphere. Strokes and other causes of damage to this region cause individuals to become functionally illiterate. They are no longer able to read **(alexia)**, write **(agraphia)**, and spell correctly. The inability to read and write is usually referred to as alexia with agraphia. Comprehension and repetition of spoken speech and the use of wrong words depends on whether the injury also involves the temporal lobe.

Memory

Memory storage functions are thought to be localized into a region called the Papez circuit, after its founder. The structures within this circuit are mostly located in the medial parts of the temporal lobes on both sides, the medial portion of the thalamus, and a structure called the fornix, a fibrous band that connects the temporal lobe and the thalamus. Several key nuclear structures within the temporal lobes called the hippocampi and the amygdaloid nuclei play an important role in the retention of memories. The hippocampi are shaped like sea horses and are located adjacent to the temporal horns of the lateral **ventricles** of the brain. The amygdaloid nuclei lie adjacent to the hippocampi and are almond shaped. Some of the structures that play a role in memory functions are in the frontal lobes. The most important of these are the cingulate gyri, which are located just above the corpus callosum on both sides of the brain. Figure 2-13 shows the hippocampus and its location.

Memory functions can be divided into three parts: registration, reinforcement and storage, and retrieval. In order to retain a piece of information, an individual must be attentive and interested in recalling the information later to initially register it in their brain. If a person is thinking about something else or daydreaming while being told something, he or she will not recall it later. The ability to recall information later is enhanced if an individual consciously tries to retain the material after it is presented. This is done by repeating the information, or by relating it to something else to reinforce it. For example one might recall a name like Blaire, which resembles your sister's name, Claire, or that rhymes with

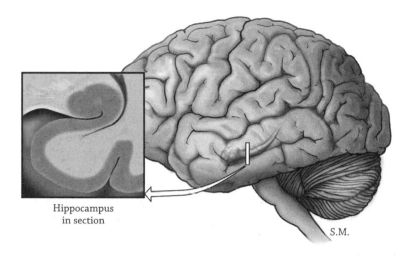

Hippocampus
in section

S.M.

FIGURE 2-13 The insert shows the hippocampus and its location as viewed from the outer aspect of the brain.

fair. Once it is reinforced and repeated, it is probably stored within structures in the Papez circuit for later retrieval. Information is most likely stored for later retrieval much like files in a filing cabinet. Later retrieval of information probably begins in the frontal lobes, which access the stored information in the Papez circuit. If I ask people who their third-grade teacher was, most of them will somehow try to access that information by imagining themselves in the school that they attended at the time. They might recall their mother sending them lunch, or the little girl in pigtails in the row next to them, or friends at school; or they may directly visualize the teacher in front of their class. Similarly, if I ask the name of a fruit, individuals will often try to visualize the fruit or recall its taste to enter their "fruit file." Patients with frontal lobe strokes and with Alzheimer's disease often have difficulty retrieving memories and ordering them chronologically. Patients with temporal lobe lesions often have difficulty with memory storage.

The left temporal lobe and thalamus are specialized for word and language memories, and the right temporal lobe and thalamus are specialized for visual memories.

Memory and language are two functions that organize and integrate the sensory and perceptual functions of the brain. Having discussed these two integrative functions and some of the various forms of perception (vision, hearing, feeling, and motor function), I will briefly discuss general patterns of cerebral hemisphere functions.

One important theme of cerebral functions is the interrelationship between motor and sensory functions. Let's use vision as an example. Suppose I show someone a picture of a scene. Most observers first see a key element within the scene. This is done in the striate visual cortex within the occipital lobes. This initial visual information then generates questions that the viewer tries to answer by looking further at the picture with their eyes. Eye movement searches are generated by the frontal lobe gaze centers. This looking induces further input of visual information (i.e., more seeing), which in turn raises further questions and stimulates more looking. Gradually the viewer gets more and more information from the picture. The process of exploration, a motor behavior that we call "looking" in the visual sphere, and a perceptual activity that we refer to as "seeing" in the visual sphere, together result in acquiring maximal information. Of course the information an individual acquires depends on their intelligence and experience. Referring to their memory zones within the temporal lobes and thalami, and referring to their language area in the left parasylvian areas, helps with the interpretation of the visual information and assignment of names to the various things that they see. If someone had never seen a giraffe, they would have difficulty identifying or naming a picture of a giraffe.

Similarly, if I blindfold you and place something in your hand, you will feel something, generate possibilities for the nature of the object, and palpate (i.e., manually explore) the object to detect its nature and its name. The tactile perception takes place in the somatosensory area within the postcentral gyrus of the parietal lobe opposite to the hand in which the object is placed, and the manual movements of exploration are generated in the hand and arm area of the precentral gyrus in the opposite frontal lobe. Similarly, if I play a tune on a piano, hearing the tune occurs in the lateral portion of the temporal lobes, at which point the individual tries to listen or tune in to certain aspects of the music. This tuning is probably a frontal lobe function. Of course as in seeing, accurate identification of the nature of the object to be felt, and the music played, depends heavily on the individual's prior experience. If they have never heard the tune or felt the object, they would not be able to identify it correctly or give it a name.

Another important theme is the connections and circuitry between perceptual regions—all located behind the central sulcus—and language and memory regions. For example, suppose I show you a familiar coffee mug. You first see the cup with your eyes and your visual cortex. Transmission of the visual data to your language area in the left cerebral hemisphere will probably result in generation of the word name *mug* or *cup*. Transmission of the information to your visual memory area in the right medial temporal lobes and then the left medial temporal lobe enables you to remember that this particular cup was given to you as a present by your office staff and that you use that mug for coffee each morning at work. Activation of the taste regions in your temporal lobes reinforces that coffee is the only substance ever placed in this mug, and the tactile zones in your parietal lobes might result in your recalling the feel of the touch of the mug in your hands in the morning and that the mug is made of clay. Relay of information between the various sensory areas, the motor exploration areas, memory, and language has allowed you to characterize the nature of that particular object.

The other element I have left out of the above discussion is the affective element of perceptions. Some of the things that we see, hear, feel, and otherwise experience have an emotional effect upon us. These perceptions somehow make us feel fearful, uneasy, happy, angry, excited, or sad. At times we are quite aware of the emotional content of the perceptions but at other times we are not. Perceptions also have a circuitry through the limbic lobes of the brain, including the temporal lobes and the cingulate gyri, that gives our observations and experiences an emotional and affective value. The right cerebral hemisphere may have more influence on the emotive, affective content than the left cerebral hemisphere.

Emotions, Affect, and Self-Image

There are both psychological and physiological changes in patients' self-image after strokes. Strokes often create deficits that are easily visible to everyone, even during casual encounters with stroke survivors. Abnormalities of facial appearance, limb use, walking, and speech are often quite obvious to all observers. Since their bodies have changed, it is quite natural and understandable that patients will worry whether or not the changes will prove acceptable and tolerable to others. This is especially problematic when the caregivers will need to alter their own activities in important ways to help the patients. Will they be willing and able to handle the new responsibility? Will the caregivers pitch in happily, or will the patient feel like an unwanted burden? Significant others must understand the worries that patients naturally have, and must try to calm and reassure the patients whenever possible.

Physiological changes due to stroke are usually in the other direction; that is, patients do not fully comprehend the nature and severity of their deficits and are inappropriately unconcerned. The right cerebral hemisphere is important in regard to both awareness of deficits and emotive responses toward them. Some individuals with large right cerebral hemisphere strokes who have left limb paralysis and loss of attention to their left visual field may completely deny that anything is wrong with them. This lack of awareness of the deficit is called anosognosia. I recall rather vividly being called to the emergency room of my hospital at 3:00 A.M. by a perplexed and desperate husband and doctor-in-training. A woman had very suddenly developed complete paralysis of her left limbs and was brought to the hospital by her husband despite her resistance. She absolutely refused to be admitted to the hospital declaring that nothing was the matter with her. Neither the husband nor any of the emergency room personnel had been able to convince her otherwise, so I was summoned. I examined her and found that she had complete left-sided paralysis, loss of sensation in her left limbs and body, and a lack of response to objects on her left side. After the examination she said, "You see, nothing is wrong with me." Rather than argue, I gave her the car keys and said that if she could walk to her car and drive home, she could go. She tried to get up and slipped to the floor, unable to rise. She accused me of tripping her, but said that now she had to stay because of her fall. Not until her second week in the hospital did she develop any realization of anything wrong with her limbs, feeling, or vision. Her stroke had affected the right frontal and parietal lobes, regions that are involved with evaluating and reacting to the left side of the body and space.

Emotive reactions are also often blunted in patients with right cerebral damage. They often have difficulty expressing emotions in their facial expressions and voices and may have difficulty picking up the body language and emotional tones of others. This abnormality of affect has been referred to as dysprosody, which literally means an abnormality of the rhythm and tone of speech. Speech has two major aspects. One is linguistic and relates strictly to the meaning of the words used. The other aspect is affective. By varying the tone, volume, accent, facial expression, gestures, and word emphasis, speakers can give the same words very different meanings. The phrase "come home early" when spoken by a spouse may have many meanings depending on how and when the words are spoken. They could mean, "If you get a chance, it would be nice if you were early." They could also mean, "You had better be home early."

The words could have a sexual or other connotation, indicating some reward for an early appearance or punishment for not arriving early. The ability to transmit and interpret body language and emotional tone of communications is an important part of communication between individuals. Strokes, especially those in the right cerebral hemisphere, can blunt affective responses and alter nonlinguistic communications. These problems should be explained to caregivers and significant others.

Chapter 3

How Does the Body Bring Blood to the Brain?

The Anatomy of the Heart and Brain-Supplying Blood Vessels

Strokes involve blockage and breakage of the blood vessels that bring blood to the brain or that lie next to and within the brain. Just as a plumber needs to know what pipes go to a malfunctioning sink and how those pipes get from the water source to that sink, doctors must try to localize the blood vessels that are blocked or leaking in order to find out what is wrong with them. When the location of the blood vessel abnormality is known, modern imaging techniques can be used to define the type of abnormality within the abnormal vessels. Identifying the location and nature of the problem in the heart and blood vessels is important for choosing treatment.

Blood is pumped from the heart into the **aorta,** the largest artery in the body. The aorta issues from the left ventricle of the heart. **Arteries** that supply the brain branch from the aorta, pass through the neck, and enter the cranium to supply blood to the brain. **Veins** drain blood from the brain, which then reenters the heart to recirculate. Strokes can be caused by many different abnormalities that affect blood vessels at any point within this heart–aorta–neck arteries–cranial arteries–veins circuit. In this chapter I will review the basic anatomy of the heart and these blood vessels. In Chapter 5 I will discuss the types of conditions that affect these vascular structures.

The Heart

The heart is divided by partitions called septa into left and right sides. Each side of the heart is further divided into an upper chamber called an **atrium,** which receives blood flow, and a **ventricle,** which pumps blood out. Figure 3-1 shows the various chambers of the heart. Valves are placed between the atria and the ventricles to control the normal flow of blood. The valves in the heart make sure that blood goes in the correct direction and not backwards from the ventricles into the atria or from the aorta or pulmonary artery back into the ventricles. After the chambers have contracted, expelling their contents, valves close behind the contractions.

The left atrium receives blood from the lungs by way of the pulmonary vein. (*Pulmonary* is a term often used to refer to the lungs). This blood has already traveled through the lungs where it has been saturated with oxygen, and so it looks red. The muscle in the left atrium contracts and sends blood through the **mitral valve** located between the left atrium and the left ventricle. The left ventricle then pumps blood through the **aortic valve** into the

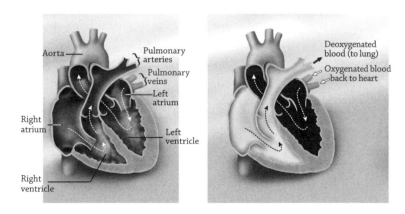

FIGURE 3-1 The heart chambers and valves.

aorta. Blood travels through arteries that branch from the aorta, including those that lead to the brain, to supply the body's organs with oxygen and nutrients. The large arteries branch into smaller arteries and then into very small vessels called arterioles and even smaller **capillaries.** At the capillary level, the blood is in close contact with the cells within the body's organs. These cells remove oxygen and nutrients from the blood. Blood then returns to the heart from the organs by way of veins. Sugar and other nutrients are added to the blood as the veins drain the intestinal tract and the liver. The largest veins are the superior vena cava, which drains blood from the upper body, and the inferior vena cava, which drains blood from structures located in the lower part of the body, those located below the diaphragm (the muscular structure that separates the chest from the abdomen). The venae cavae empty blood into the right atrium. This blood looks blue since most of the oxygen has been removed.

The right atrium contracts, pushing blood through the **tricuspid valve** located between the right atrium and right ventricle. Contraction of the right ventricular heart muscle ejects blood through the **pulmonary valve** into the **pulmonary artery,** which leads to the lungs. This artery divides into two branches that supply the left and right lungs. In the lungs the blood is oxygenated. The redder-looking oxygenated blood then travels via the pulmonary veins back to the left atrium where the circuit begins again. Figure 3-1 shows the various heart structures described.

The Aorta and Its Main Brain-Supplying Branches

The aorta gives rise to arteries that supply the brain with needed energy and oxygen. The branches of the aorta are diagrammed

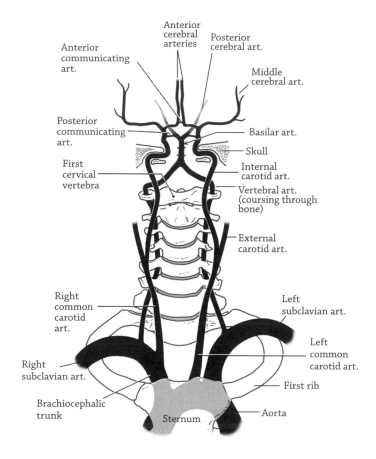

FIGURE 3-2a Arteries branching from the aorta that lead into the neck and head.

in Figure 3-2a. The first branch arising from the right side of the aortic arch is the brachiocephalic trunk, which is also called the innominate artery. This vessel then branches into the right subclavian artery, which runs under the clavicle to supply blood to the right arm, and the common carotid artery, which branches to supply the right face and neck (the right external carotid artery) and the front portion of the right cerebral hemisphere and the right eye (the right internal carotid artery). The right subclavian artery gives rise to the right vertebral artery, which supplies the right medulla and lower back portion of the right cerebellum, and then joins with the left vertebral artery inside the skull. The next branch from the aortic arch is the left common carotid artery, which supplies the left face and neck (the left external carotid artery) and the front portion of the left cerebral hemisphere and the left eye (left internal carotid artery). The last branch is the left subclavian artery, which gives rise to the left vertebral artery, which supplies the left medulla and lower back portion of the left cerebellum, and then joins with the right vertebral artery to supply the remainder of the brainstem and cerebellum and back portion of the cerebral hemispheres.

Arteries within the Neck

Figure 3-2b is a drawing of the neck that shows the anatomy of the right carotid arteries and the right vertebral arteries. The right common carotid artery divides high in the neck into the right external carotid artery (which gives branches to the structures in the face and structures within the head other than the brain, such as the nose and mouth) and the internal carotid artery (which supplies the right eye and the major portion of the right cerebrum). The right vertebral artery courses through the vertebral column and then enters the back of the head through a hole in the back of the skull (the **foramen** magnum). The left carotid and vertebral arteries supply the comparable left-sided structures. Figure 3-2a shows the paths of the right- and left-sided arteries in a frontal view of the body.

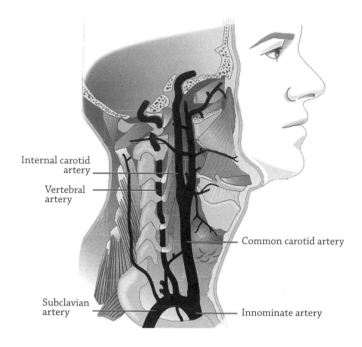

Internal carotid artery

Vertebral artery

Common carotid artery

Subclavian artery

Innominate artery

FIGURE 3-2b Arteries on the right side of the neck. From *Caplan's Stroke: A Clinical Approach,* 4th ed., Philadelphia, Saunders-Elsevier, 2009, with permission.

Arteries within the Skull

Inside the skull, each internal carotid artery divides into a middle cerebral artery, which supplies mostly the structures on the outer lateral surface of the cerebral hemispheres; and an anterior cerebral artery, which supplies the brain structures near the midline. Figure 3-3a shows the branching of the right middle cerebral artery on the lateral surface of the brain. The medial aspect of the brain is shown in Figure 3-3b. This shows the distribution of the anterior cerebral artery. The back portion of the cerebral hemispheres is supplied by the posterior cerebral arteries, which branch from the basilar artery.

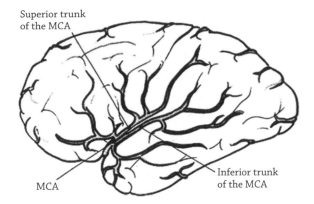

FIGURE 3-3a Right middle cerebral artery (MCA) branches on the lateral surface of the brain. From *Caplan's Stroke: A Clinical Approach,* 3rd ed., Boston, Butterworth-Heinemann, 2000, with permission.

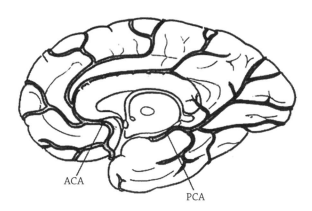

FIGURE 3-3b Arterial branches of the anterior cerebral artery (ACA) and posterior cerebral artery (PCA) on the medial surface of the brain. From *Caplan's Stroke: A Clinical Approach,* 3rd ed., Boston, Butterworth-Heinemann, 2000, with permission.

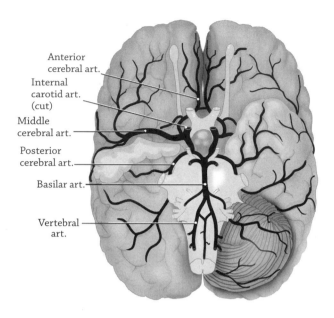

Anterior
cerebral art.
Internal
carotid art.
(cut)
Middle
cerebral art.
Posterior
cerebral art.
Basilar art.
Vertebral
art.

FIGURE 3-3c Arteries on the undersurface of the brain and their supply.

The posterior cerebral artery supply on the medial portion of the cerebral hemispheres is shown on Figure 3-3b and on the inferior surface of the brain in Figure 3-3c. Figure 3-4 is a drawing of an arteriogram that shows the branching of the right internal carotid artery.

The parts of the brain not supplied by the internal carotid arteries are nourished through the two vertebral arteries that ascend toward the brain in the back of the neck on each side. They are called *vertebral* because they travel through the bony vertebral column. The two vertebral arteries supply the medulla oblongata and the back undersurface of the cerebellum on each side and then join to form the basilar artery, a midline blood vessel that supplies the brainstem above the medulla oblongata on both sides (see Figures 3-2a and 3-3c). Near its termination, the basilar artery gives off

(a)

(b)

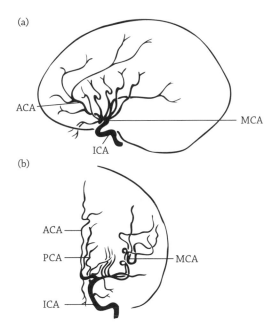

FIGURE 3-4 Drawing of carotid angiograms (lateral view in a, anteroposterior view in b). ICA= internal carotid artery, MCA = middle cerebral artery, ACA= anterior cerebral artery, PCA= posterior cerebral artery. From From *Caplan's Stroke: A Clinical Approach,* 3rd ed., Boston, Butterworth-Heinemann, 2000, with permission.

branches that supply the upper surface of the cerebellum on both sides. The basilar artery divides at a midbrain level and gives off branches to the thalami and to the temporal and occipital lobes of the cerebral hemispheres on each side. The ending, large-artery branches of the basilar artery are termed the posterior cerebral arteries.

The large arteries give off successively smaller branches called arterioles and capillaries. Some of these small arterial branches are shown in Figure 3-5, a picture of the brain after the blood vessels have been injected with dye. Arrows point to some of the very small

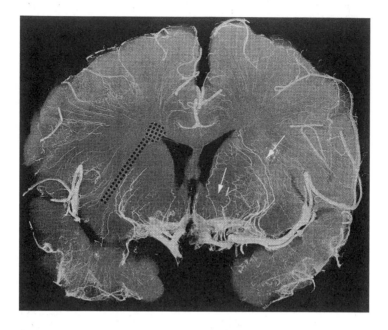

FIGURE 3-5 Postmortem angiogram showing branches of the cerebral arteries. From Pullicino P, "Lenticulostriate Arteries," in Bogousslavsky J, Caplan LR, eds., *Stroke Syndromes,* 2nd ed., Cambridge, England: Cambridge University Press, 2001, with permission.

arterial branches that are visible. The smallest arterial branches are minute and are only able to be seen through a microscope.

Veins

Veins are located deep within the brain and on its surface. These veins drain into large venous structures, the **dural venous sinuses**, located within layers of the **dura mater,** the hard membrane that surrounds the brain and is located just beneath the skull. From the dural sinuses, blood drains into large neck veins, and from there into the heart. The largest neck veins are called the jugular

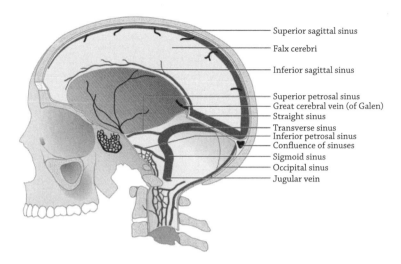

FIGURE 3-6 Side view of the brain and neck showing some of the main venous structures. From *Caplan's Stroke: A Clinical Approach,* 4th ed., Philadelphia, Saunders- Elsevier, 2009, with permission.

veins. Figure 3-6 is a drawing of the side of the head and neck that shows the location of some of the major veins. When veins become blocked, blood and fluid cannot easily drain from the head, and water builds up within the brain regions that are drained by the blocked veins.

Chapter 4

What Is a Stroke? What Are the Different Kinds of Stroke?

After discussing what the brain looks like, how it works, and how it is supplied with blood, I now turn to discussing the various types of stroke and how they affect the brain and the blood vessels that supply it. I will discuss the various medical conditions and causes of the different types of stroke in Chapter 5. In order for readers to understand how they might try to prevent stroke, what conditions doctors look for in order to prevent strokes from happening, how they evaluate patients with stroke, and how they treat stroke patients, it is clearly necessary to understand something about stroke. So, key questions that are important to ask are: What is a stroke? What are its causes? What are the risk factors that predispose to stroke? I will try to concisely answer these queries in this chapter.

What is a stroke?

The brain, like every other organ in the body, depends on a constant supply of energy to function normally. The brain's fuel is carried in the blood. The two main energy sources that the brain uses for energy and function are sugar and oxygen. Oxygen is carried mainly in the hemoglobin of red blood cells, and sugar is carried in the serum of the blood. When a part of the brain is not supplied with an adequate supply of blood, or when the blood does not carry enough oxygen or sugar, that portion of the brain becomes unable to perform its normal functions. When a brain area stops working, the function that was located in that area ceases at least until energy is restored. So if blood is not delivered normally to the region in the left hemisphere that subserves speech, then speech will be lost or become abnormal.

Stroke is a term used to describe brain injury caused by an abnormality of the blood supply to a part of the brain. The word is derived from the fact that most stroke patients are stricken suddenly by the blood vessel abnormality, and abnormalities of brain function begin quickly, sometimes within an instant.

Stroke is a very broad term that describes a variety of different types of conditions that involve the blood vessels that supply the brain with needed nourishment and fuel. Since treatment depends on the type of stroke and the location of the blood vessels involved, it is very important for treating doctors to determine precisely what caused the vascular and brain injury and where the abnormalities are located.

What Are the Different Types of Strokes?

Strokes can be divided into two very broad groups: hemorrhage and ischemia. Hemorrhage refers to bleeding inside the skull, either into the brain or into the fluid surrounding the brain. Ischemia refers to a lack of blood (*-emia* is a suffix that means having a particular blood condition or something in the blood). Hemorrhage and ischemia are polar opposites. Hemorrhage is characterized by too much blood inside the skull, ischemia means there is not enough of a blood supply to allow continued normal functioning of the affected brain tissue. Brain ischemia is much more common than hemorrhage; about four strokes out of every five are ischemic.

Hemorrhage

There are several different subtypes of hemorrhage. These are named for their locations inside of the skull. The brain is surrounded by three membranes; from the innermost, toward the skull, they are

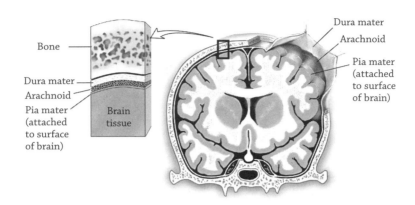

FIGURE 4-1 The membranes around the brain.

called the pia mater, **arachnoid**, and dura mater. These names come from Latin. Pia mater means "soft mother"; this inner membrane is thin and covers the brain a bit like plastic cling wrap. Arachnoid means like a small insect; this name was given from the observation that this middle membrane is a bit like a spider web. The outer membrane is firm and more substantial than the others and is called the dura mater, literally meaning "hard mother." These layers are shown in Figure 4-1. Hemorrhages within the brain substance (inside the pia mater) are called intracerebral hemorrhages; those between the pia mater and arachnoid are labeled subarachnoid hemorrhages. Hemorrhages outside of the arachnoid but inside of the dura mater are called subdural hemorrhages, and hemorrhages outside of the dura mater but inside of the skull are called epidural hemorrhages. These sites of bleeding are shown in Figure 4-2. The different sites of bleeding have different causes.

Bleeding into the brain is referred to as intracerebral hemorrhage, *intracerebral* meaning into the cerebrum (another term often used for the brain). Bleeding into the brain tears and disconnects vital nerve centers and pathways. The bleeding is due

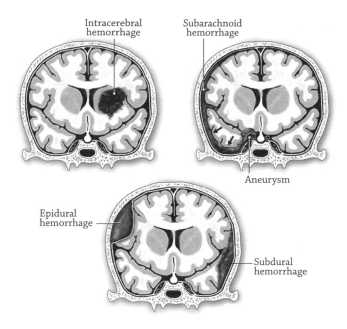

FIGURE 4-2 Examples of intracerebral, subarachnoid, subdural, and epidural hemorrhages.

to rupture of small blood vessels, the arterioles and capillaries within the brain substance. The bleeding in patients with intracerebral hemorrhage is most often due to uncontrolled hypertension. Other less common causes are listed in Table 4-1. The blood usually oozes into the brain under pressure and forms a localized, often round or elliptical blood collection called a hematoma. The hematoma separates normal brain structures and interrupts brain pathways called tracts. Hematomas also exert pressure on brain regions adjacent to the collected blood and can injure these tissues. Large hemorrhages are often fatal because they increase pressure within the skull, squeezing vital regions within the brainstem. Bleeding into the fluid around the brain is called subarachnoid hemorrhage, a term chosen since the blood collects and

TABLE 4-1 Most common causes of hemorrhages by their most frequent sites

Intracerebral hemorrhages
   Hypertension
   Abnormal bleeding functions
   Prescribed anticoagulants like warfarin, dabigatran, apixaban
   Low platelet count (thrombocytopenia)
   Bleeding tendencies like hemophilia
   After receiving thrombolytic drugs
   Vascular malformations
   Amyloids within blood vessels in the brain
   Trauma
   Bleeding into brain tumors and brain infarcts
Subarachnoid hemorrhages
   Arterial aneurysms
   Vascular malformations near the brain surface
   Bleeding tendencies
   Head injury
Subdural hemorrhages
   Trauma
   Bleeding tendencies
Epidural hemorrhages
   Trauma

stays under the arachnoid membrane that lies over the pia mater. Subarachnoid hemorrhages are usually caused by rupture of an aneurysm, a weakened artery whose wall is ballooned outward. The artery breaks, spilling blood instantly into the fluid that circulates around the brain and spinal cord. The sudden release of blood under high pressure increases the pressure inside the skull and causes severe, sudden-onset headache, often with vomiting. The abrupt increase in pressure causes a lapse in brain function; afflicted patients may stare, drop to their knees, or become confused and unable to remember.

The symptoms in patients with subarachnoid hemorrhage most often relate to diffuse abnormalities of brain function, since usually there is no bleeding into just one part of the brain. By contrast, in patients with intracerebral hemorrhages, the hematoma is localized and causes loss of function related to the area damaged by the local blood collection. For example, if the bleeding is into the left cerebral hemisphere, the patient often has weakness and loss of feeling in the right limbs and a loss of normal speech. A hemorrhage into the cerebellum will cause dizziness and a loss of balance. Tom M., the third patient introduced in Chapter 1, had an intracerebral hemorrhage in his left cerebellum. Recall that he suddenly became dizzy, staggered, and vomited. He was also unable to walk. The cerebellum is specialized for balance, equilibrium, and coordination in walking. The cerebellar hemorrhage had formed a very well circumscribed hematoma (much like the upper left drawing in Figure 4-2) that had disrupted important functions related to balance. The particular symptoms that patients with intracerebral hemorrhages develop relate to the region of bleeding and are described as focal—that is, related to dysfunction of only one brain region, such as the left cerebellum in the case of Tom M. In subarachnoid hemorrhage, the symptoms are diffuse and not localized to one area.

Subdural and epidural hemorrhages are most often caused by head injuries that tear blood vessels. In subdural hemorrhages the bleeding is usually from veins that lie within the space between the arachnoid membrane and the dura mater. In epidural hemorrhages the bleeding most often results from tearing of meningeal arteries. Often there is an accompanying skull fracture that has torn a meningeal artery. Blood accumulates much faster when it issues from arteries than it does from small veins, so that symptoms usually develop soon after head injury in patients with epidural hemorrhages. In subdural hemorrhages the bleeding can be slow so that symptoms of headache and brain dysfunction may be delayed for weeks after the head injury.

The most common causes of hemorrhages at the various sites are listed in Table 4-1 (the most important are in bold). The skull forms a closed hard sphere, a fortress around the brain and its surrounding membranes, but the fortress can become a prison that limits the exit of blood from within the skull. The closed system means that the bleeding causes pressure to build up quickly and strangle normal tissues by compressing them.

Brain Ischemia

A decrease of blood supply to the brain is called *ischemia*. If the ischemia is prolonged enough it leads to the death of tissue, called infarction.

There are three different major categories of brain ischemia, each indicating a different mechanism of blood vessel injury or reason for decreased blood flow. These three categories are often referred to as thrombosis, embolism, and systemic hypoperfusion. Figure 4-3 illustrates these different mechanisms of ischemia. I find it is easiest for laypeople to understand these terms by using a familiar analogy to house plumbing. Suppose that one morning when you turn on the faucet in the children's bathroom on the second floor, no water comes out, or instead water only dribbles out weakly. The malfunctioning sink could be due to a local problem, such as rust buildup in the pipe leading to that sink. This type of problem is analogous to thrombosis, a term used to describe a local problem that involves a blood vessel, an artery, that supplies the brain. Atherosclerosis or another type of disease often narrows the blood-flow channel (the **lumen**) of the artery. When the lumen becomes very narrow, blood flow is severely reduced, causing localized stagnation of the blood column. This change in flow causes blood to clot, resulting in total occlusion of the artery. Clearly this is a local problem in one pipe; a plumber would approach this problem by attempting to fix the damaged blocked pipe. Similarly treating physicians could treat a narrowed (stenosed) or occluded artery by trying to open it or by

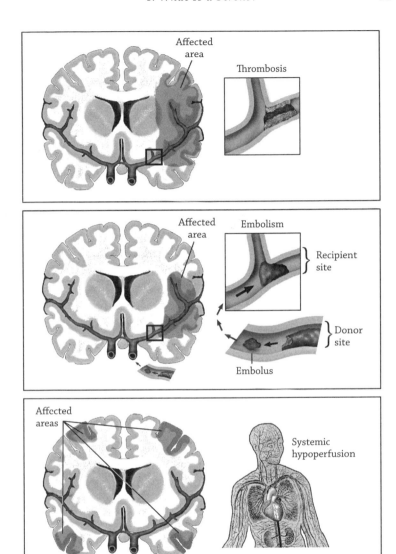

FIGURE 4-3 The different types of ischemic stroke: thrombosis, embolism, and systemic hypoperfusion.

creating a detour around it. Robert H., the first patient introduced in Chapter 1, had a stroke due to thrombosis of his right internal carotid artery in the neck. The cause was chronic atherosclerosis that had gradually developed in that and other arteries. I will discuss in later chapters how doctors were able to show the nature of his problem and how they treated him.

Alternatively, blockage of the pipe to that second-floor sink could have been due to debris in the water system that happened by chance to come to rest in that pipe, rather than being due to a local problem that began within the pipe. An artery within the head or neck that supplies the brain can be blocked by a blood clot or other particulate matter that breaks loose from a downstream site. The source could be from one of three locations: the heart, the aorta (the major artery leading away from the heart), or from one of the major arteries in the neck located before the blockage but along the same circulatory pathway. The process of particles breaking loose and blocking a distant artery is referred to as embolism. The source of the material is called the donor site and the receiving vessel is called the recipient site; the material itself is called an embolus. Robert H. had an embolus break off from the thrombus that had developed in his right carotid artery. The embolus traveled into his head and blocked his right middle cerebral artery. Elaine S., the fourth patient introduced in Chapter 1, had an embolus that arose in her fibrillating left atrium and that traveled to her right middle cerebral artery, causing her left limbs to suddenly become weak. By contrast, Claire H. had a tear in her left carotid artery in the neck. Clot material that formed in that artery embolized to her left middle cerebral artery, suddenly rendering her speechless and her right arms and legs weak. Embolism is the most common cause of ischemic strokes. I will say much more later in the book about how doctors diagnose embolism and choose treatment.

A third reason for poor flow in the second-floor sink might be a general problem with the water tank, water pump, or water pressure. In that case, flow through all the sinks and baths in the house should be affected. Simply turning on the faucet in other sinks in the house will reveal the nature of the problem. Water should also flow poorly in the other sinks and showers. In the body, this type of problem is referred to as systemic hypoperfusion. Abnormal performance of the pump (heart) could lead to low pressure in the system. Abnormally slow or fast heart rhythms, cardiac arrest, and failure of the heart to pump blood adequately can all lead to diminished blood flow to the head and brain. Other causes of diminished circulatory functions are a lowering of blood pressure and blood flow due to an inadequate amount of blood and fluid in the vascular compartment of the body. Bleeding, dehydration, and loss of fluid into body tissues (shock) can all lead to inadequate brain perfusion. This would be akin to having an empty or very low water tank. The cartoons in Figure 4-4 illustrate the plumbing analogy.

In patients with brain embolism and thrombosis, one artery is usually blocked, leading to dysfunction of the part of the brain supplied by that blocked artery. This shows itself by focal abnormalities of brain function, such as weakness of the limbs on one side of the body. In this respect the abnormalities are similar to those found in patients with local brain hematomas. By contrast, systemic hypoperfusion leads to more diffuse abnormalities such as light-headedness, dizziness, confusion, and dimming of vision or hearing. Patients look pale and are generally weak. These symptoms are caused by a generalized reduction in blood flow and not by loss of function in one local region of the brain.

The importance of differentiating the types of ischemia should appear obvious. If we return to the plumbing analogy, a local problem in one pipe (thrombosis) could be potentially fixed by work only on that pipe. If, however, the problem is caused by temporary blockage of that same pipe by loose matter in the system, then removing the blockage in the occluded pipe would likely be followed by another pipe being blocked later by the same problem. Somehow the particles must be removed from the system and their subsequent formation need to be prevented if possible. If the problem is

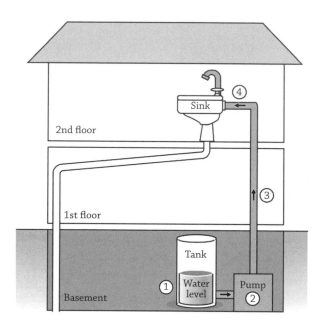

FIGURE 4-4 Plumbing diagram.

in the pump or tank, or with the water pressure in general, then no work on a single pipe will be helpful.

By definition, brain ischemia refers to an inadequate supply of blood to a part of the brain. Arteries bring to the brain oxygen, sugar, and other nutrients necessary for survival. An analogy would be a yard with grass or a vegetable garden. If water and sun are inadequate and the ground does not get enough nourishment, the grass and vegetables will eventually die. Before the grass dies it often appears brown, but watering it may restore its normal green color and appearance. Similarly, if the lack of blood flow is brief or relatively minor in degree, there may be temporary loss of function during the brief period of ischemia, but function may return to normal when blood flow is restored. Temporary decreases in blood flow to a part of the brain are often referred to as transient ischemic attacks (TIAs). They are caused by temporary blockage of an artery by an embolus that then passes, or temporary inadequacy of blood flow through a narrowed artery. These temporary attacks indicate that something is wrong with the system, and so warn of the possibility of a stroke.

Recall that Robert H. had several TIAs before his stroke. In one brief episode, his left hand and arm went numb. In another attack, his left face and hand tingled. These spells indicated temporary decrease in blood flow to a portion of his right cerebral hemisphere, which controls movement and feeling in his left face, arm, and hand. In yet another episode, he temporarily lost vision in his right eye. This indicated a transient decrease in blood flow to that eye. The right eye and the right cerebral hemisphere are supplied with blood by the right internal carotid artery. These episodes indicated that blood flow was a problem in that artery, but unfortunately Robert H. and his doctors did not attend to this problem before he developed a severe stroke due to total blockage of his right internal carotid artery.

Having discussed the way that abnormalities of the blood and blood flow cause brain injury and strokes, in the next chapter I will discuss the types of medical conditions that cause strokes and TIAs.

Chapter 5

What Are the Medical Conditions That Cause Strokes?

Abnormalities of three major body components explain the development of strokes: (1) the heart, (2) the blood vessels that supply and drain the brain, and (3) the blood. Often changes occur in more than one of these components. In many patients who have abnormalities involving the heart or the blood vessels, changes in the blood (e.g., an increased tendency to clot) can explain why a stroke develops at a particular time. The anatomy of the heart and blood vessels was discussed in Chapter 3. This chapter discusses the abnormalities (pathology) in these structures that lead to strokes. Blood and its pathology will also be introduced and discussed.

Blood Vessels

To understand the various conditions that affect blood vessels, it is necessary to know something of the composition and function of the arteries that bring blood to the brain and the veins that drain blood from the brain.

Arteries contain three layers: an inner, relatively thin **intima** coat that contains an inner membrane called the endothelium, a central **media** coat that is composed of smooth muscle and elastic and connective tissue, and an outer coat called the **adventitia**. Figure 5-1 shows the different layers within normal arteries. The

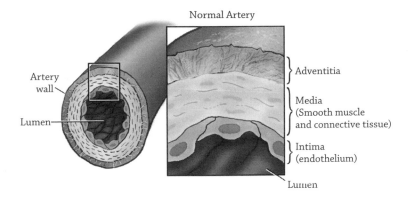

Normal Artery

Artery wall

Lumen

Adventitia

Media
(Smooth muscle
and connective tissue)

Intima
(endothelium)

Lumen

FIGURE 5-1 Cross section of a normal artery showing the various coats.

inner coat is lined by endothelium, which forms a barrier between the blood in the center of the artery (the lumen) and the wall of the artery. The flexibility and the capacity for muscular contraction within the medial coat gives the artery the ability to narrow (constrict) or widen (dilate), allowing it to change capacity as needed by the organ that it supplies with blood.

Arteries bring blood to the brain. Veins in and on the surface of the brain and within the dura mater drain blood away from the brain. Veins are thinner walled than arteries and do not have a muscular coat. Blood drained from the brain enters the right atrium, then is pumped by the right ventricle to the lungs where it will pick up oxygen. The passage of blood to and from the lungs is called **pulmonary circulation.** Blood goes from the lungs back to the left side of the heart, where it will again be pumped to the aorta and to the **systemic circulation** (body organs other than the lungs) arteries.

Blood Vessel Abnormalities That Cause Brain Ischemia and Infarction

Atherosclerosis (Arteriosclerosis)

Degenerative changes in the arteries that supply blood to vital organs develop to some extent in all of us if we live long enough. This degeneration is most often referred to as **atherosclerosis** (*athero* referring to fatty accumulations, and *sclerosis* to hardening). **Arteriosclerosis** (literally, hardening of arteries) is another common term used. This degeneration is characterized by the development of plaques on the inside of arteries, and wear and tear affecting the wall of the arteries, leading to decreased elasticity and stiffness of the arteries. Atherosclerotic plaques (atheromas) develop in the aorta and in the large arteries in the neck and head that supply the brain with blood.

The earliest atherosclerotic abnormalities are called fatty streaks, which are visible as regions of yellowish discoloration of the intima of the aorta and the large and medium-sized systemic and cerebrovascular arteries. Fatty streaks begin to develop in childhood. The fat comes from fatty substances (lipids) within the blood. The lipids are deposited within and outside of cells and accumulate along with smooth muscle cells, beneath the intima to form these fatty streaks. Later in life, firm (fibrous) plaques develop in the same regions as these fatty streaks. These plaques consist of lipids, smooth muscle, fibrous and connective tissue, white blood cells, and crystals of cholesterol. Some plaques are soft, while others are very firm and even calcified.

When atherosclerotic plaques enlarge, they narrow the lumen of the artery and so decrease blood flow and cause changes in the bloodstream, often with turbulence. Figure 5-2 shows a large plaque that encroaches on the lumen of an artery. The irregular surface of the plaque attracts small structures within the blood called platelets. These stick to each other and form bonds with fibrin, a protein formed

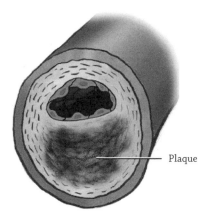

FIGURE 5-2 Large atherosclerotic plaque narrowing an artery.

in the blood from **fibrinogen.** These platelet-fibrin clumps are white and so are often called white clots. They stick to each other and to the rough regions on the surface of the plaques (see Figure 5-3). In addition, cracks in the plaques activate clotting factors in the blood. Red blood cells form a mesh with fibrin; these clots derive their color from the red blood cells and so are often called red clots.

Atherosclerotic large-artery abnormalities cause ischemia in three major ways:

1. Severe luminal narrowing markedly decreases blood flow leading to brain ischemia in the territory of the compromised artery (hypoperfusion).
2. Plaques or occlusive thrombi mechanically block branches of the main arteries, leading to hypoperfusion in the distribution of these branches of the artery.
3. Propagation and embolization of thrombi cause occlusion of distal branches. Emboli can consist of red thrombi, white platelet–fibrin aggregates, or elements of plaques such as cholesterol crystals.

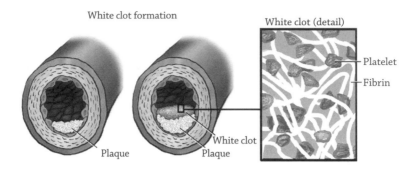

FIGURE 5-3 Plaque forming in an artery and white platelet–fibrin thrombus attached to the plaque. The insert shows a white clot as it looks under a microscope.

Robert H., the first patient described in Chapter 1, had an atherosclerotic plaque in his right internal carotid artery in the neck. When the plaque narrowed the artery, small particles broke off and caused his TIAs. The severe narrowing of the artery slowed blood flow and allowed a red clot to form and totally occlude the artery. A large part of this red clot broke off and moved into his head (embolized) and caused his stroke. He also had atherosclerotic damage to the coronary arteries in his heart and in the arteries that supply blood to his legs.

Many conditions promote and accelerate the development of atherosclerotic plaques. These include hypertension (especially if not well controlled), cigarette smoking, high blood cholesterol levels (elevated low-density lipoproteins [LDL] and lower high-density lipoproteins [HDL]), diabetes (especially if not well controlled), and metabolic syndrome. I will say much more about these conditions when I discuss risk factors and prevention in Chapter 8.

Hypertension

High blood pressure (hypertension) leads to wear and tear on arteries. Picture again a plumbing situation in which the water pressure is quite high. The pipes would rust and the walls of the pipes might thin with time. High blood pressure accelerates the development of atherosclerotic changes in the large arteries of the neck and head. Plaque development is more severe and occurs earlier in life than when blood pressure remains normal. Hypertension also leads to thickening of the walls of small arteries within the brain. This thickening narrows the lumen of the arteries and can lead to infarcts deep within the brain. Furthermore, hypertension can lead to a rupture of small arteries within the brain (described further in the Conditions That Cause Brain and Subarachnoid Hemorrhage section of this chapter). When uncontrolled, hypertension is the single most important risk for brain ischemia and brain hemorrhage.

Arterial Dissection

The term dissection refers to a tear in an artery. Sudden movements and stretching, as well as direct injury, can cause the wall of an artery to tear. Portions of the neck arteries that supply the brain are anchored in the neck and where they pass into the skull. Other portions of these arteries are quite mobile and can be stretched and torn. When a tear occurs, it causes bleeding within the arterial wall. The wall swells and may block blood flow in the lumen of the artery. The clot that forms within the arterial wall can be discharged into the lumen and from there embolize into the brain. Arteries within the skull can also be torn, causing brain infarction or subarachnoid hemorrhage. Dissections are a very important cause of stroke in children and young adults. They are also an important complication of neck manipulation. Figure 5-4 shows a dissection within the wall of an artery. Claire H., the

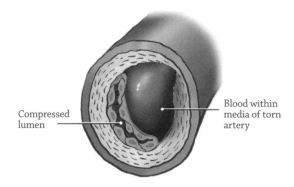

Compressed lumen

Blood within media of torn artery

FIGURE 5-4   A hematoma within the arterial wall caused by dissection of the artery.

second patient described in Chapter 1, had a dissection develop in her left internal carotid artery in the neck. The tear probably originated during vigorous sports activity.

Fibromuscular Dysplasia

This uncommon condition involves the wall of the artery. There is an excess amount of smooth muscle and connective tissue in the arterial wall, which can narrow the arterial lumen when the excess smooth muscle contracts. This vasoconstriction can block blood flow to the brain, causing infarction. It is more common in women. This disorder also can involve the arteries to the kidneys (the renal arteries), causing hypertension. Individuals with fibromuscular dysplasia have a higher than normal frequency of also harboring aneurysms in the arteries within the skull.

Arterial Dolichoectasia

Some blood vessels that supply the brain can become quite elongated and dilated and follow a tortuous and winding course with frequent loops and curves. The most common medical term used for this type of abnormality is **dolichoectasia**. The term comes from the Greek words *dolichos* (elongation) and *ectasia* (dilatation). The abnormality can involve the arteries within the neck or the skull; often both are elongated and tortuous. The widening and lengthening of the arteries can slow blood flow. In some patients blood even backs up and temporarily flows down the blood vessels back toward the heart. The elongation can distort the orifices of branches, and the slowing of blood can stimulate blood clotting within the arteries. TIAs and minor strokes are common; occasionally the arteries break and lead to subarachnoid bleeding. Dolichoectasia is caused by abnormalities in the medial and elastic coats of the arteries.

Heart and Aortic Conditions That Cause Brain Ischemia and Infarction

Blood clots and other particles can be released into the bloodstream from the heart and aorta. These particles are carried within the flowing blood toward the brain and to other organs. A familiar sight is a boat being carried vigorously downstream by a rapidly flowing river. Similarly, the particles are driven onward within the blood vessels by the force of the contractions of the heart and the blood pressure within the arteries. Arteries become smaller as they reach the organs that they supply, especially after they branch. Depending on their size and makeup, particles can get stuck at branch points or where the arterial passage in which they flow is smaller than the embolic material (see Figure 4-3, middle drawing). Blockage of the artery deprives the brain tissue it supplies of blood and nutrition. This blockage can be temporary if the embolic material breaks up and slips through the choke point. If the obstruction to blood flow lasts long enough, the brain becomes infarcted.

A number of different heart conditions and diseases lead to brain embolism. Table 5-1 lists the types of heart abnormalities that can

TABLE 5-1 Cardiac Sources of Emboli

1. Coronary artery disease and myocardial infarction
2. Arrhythmias
   Atrial fibrillation
   Sick sinus syndrome
3. Heart failure
4. Valvular heart disease
   Rheumatic (especially mitral stenosis and insufficiency)
   Mitral annulus calcification
   Mitral valve prolapse
   Calcific aortic stenosis
   Bacterial endocarditis
   Nonbacterial thrombotic endocarditis
5. Myocardiopathies
   Alcoholic cardiomyopathy
   Cocaine cardiomyopathy
   Peripartum myocardiopathy
   Myocarditis
   Sarcoidosis
   Fabry disease
   Amyloidosis
6. Cardiac tumors
   Myxomas
   Fibroelastomas
7. Septal abnormalities (paradoxical embolism)
   Atrial septal defects
   Patent foramen ovale
   Atrial septal aneurysms

lead to embolism to the brain. I discussed the anatomy and functions of the heart in Chapter 3. Clots can form in the atria or ventricles. Clots within the left atrium and left ventricle can be expelled and travel to the brain and other systemic organs.

Atrial fibrillation is a very common condition that becomes even more common as people age. About one in every 200 individuals has atrial fibrillation. As many as 5 percent of individuals over age 60 have atrial fibrillation. Atrial fibrillation describes inefficient, irregular contractions of the atria. The atria become dilated, and blood can pool within them because of the inefficient contractions. The pooling of blood leads to stagnation and the formation of red clots within the atria and the atrial appendage. These clots can then pass into the ventricles and from there into the aorta and the arteries feeding the brain and other organs. Elaine S. developed atrial fibrillation in her eighties. This condition proved to be the cause of her stroke. A clot formed in the fibrillating left atrium of her heart and embolized to her brain.

Myocardial infarctions (heart attacks) are another common source of brain embolism. Atherosclerosis, described earlier as a very important cause of brain ischemia and infarction, is the most important cause of heart ischemia and infarction. Atherosclerotic plaques within the **coronary arteries** that supply the muscle (**myocardium**) of the heart become blocked with plaques. Blockage of these arteries leads to infarction of portions of the heart muscle. The damage can lead to poor heart muscle contractility (hypokinesis) and even formation of bulges and outpouches within the ventricles (ventricular aneurysms). This damage to the heart muscle leads to depositing of clots within the interior of the heart, which can then be pumped into the aorta and bloodstream.

Brain embolism is also a major risk in patients who develop **congestive heart failure.** In this condition, the heart cannot pump out the blood that is brought into it. Blood pools in the ventricles and can clot. Coronary artery disease and hypertension are the most frequent causes of heart failure, but other, less common conditions that affect the myocardium can also lead to heart failure and brain embolism.

Various inflammatory conditions (myocarditis) and a variety of other disorders (myocardopathies) that affect the heart muscle can cause poor pumping function similar to myocardial infarction, and so also predispose a patient to clots forming within the heart and later embolizing to the brain.

Valvular Heart Disease

The heart valves can also be the site of disease that leads to brain embolism. The valves within the heart serve very important functions. They open to allow blood to flow in the desired direction and then close to prevent blood from flowing backward. **Valvular heart disease** can cause hardening of the valves, which can impair mobility and narrow the space available for blood to flow. This is called valvular stenosis. When a valve fails to close efficiently allowing backflow, the condition is called valvular insufficiency.

Rheumatic fever was once the major cause of heart valve inflammation and disease. Although the frequency of rheumatic fever and rheumatic heart disease is decreasing, it is still an important cause of heart disease. This condition often affects the mitral and aortic valves, causing **mitral insufficiency** and **mitral stenosis. Aortic stenosis** and **aortic insufficiency** are also common. Some children are born with abnormal heart valves. Aging can also lead to degenerative changes within the valves. One relatively common valve condition that is especially frequent in women is called **mitral valve prolapse,** in which portions of the mitral valve go backward into the atrium instead of going entirely into the left ventricle. Mucoid material can be deposited within the mitral valve to cause this abnormal functioning. Heart valves can also be damaged by infection. This is usually termed bacterial **endocarditis.** Some patients with cancer and other debilitating disease develop deposits of fibrin and fibrous vegetations on their heart valves. This condition is called nonbacterial thrombotic endocarditis. Valvular diseases can lead to the discharge of a number of different types of particles into the bloodstream; white and red blood clots, pieces of calcium, bacteria, and fibers that collect along the valve.

Congenital Heart Disease

Some heart problems are congenital, meaning that the defects are present at birth and remain. In some patients holes exist between the left and right atria or ventricles. These are referred to as atrial or ventricular septal defects. For many reasons, an individual can develop a blood clot (thrombus) in a vein somewhere in the body, especially in a leg vein. Sitting for a long time in one position, compressing the veins by crossing the legs, abnormal leg veins, and abnormally increased tendency for blood clotting are just some of the reasons for leg vein thrombosis. When the clot first forms, it can break loose and go to the heart with the returning venous blood. These clots most often go into the right atrium, through the tricuspid valve into the right ventricle and then through the pulmonary arteries into the lungs; this condition is called **pulmonary embolism** and can be very serious. When there is a hole between the two atria (an atrial septal defect), a thrombus formed in the leg veins reaching the right atrium can pass through the hole into the left atrium and then through the mitral valve into the left ventricle. From there the clot goes through the aortic valve into the aorta and finally into one of its systemic branches. If it enters one of the arteries to the brain, the embolus can cause a brain infarct. When defects cause clots to pass between the two circulations because of defects, it is termed paradoxical embolism, a medical term for a stroke caused this way.

Since babies' lungs do not function and do not breathe air before birth, a hole in the wall that separates the left and right fetal atria allows blood to go through the mother's circulatory system for oxygenation. At birth this oval-shaped hole, called the **foramen ovale,** a Latin phrase meaning "oval window," usually closes but, in about 30 percent of individuals, it does not fully close. When the hole remains open it is usually referred to as a **patent foramen ovale** (PFO). Figure 5-5 shows the atrial septum and defects within it.

The aorta is the largest artery within the body. The arteries that supply the brain arise from the beginning portion of the aorta within the chest. This part of the aorta and the aorta within the abdomen are regions in which atherosclerosis is often very severe.

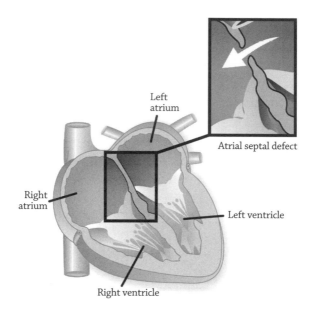

Left
atrium

Atrial septal defect

Right
atrium

Left ventricle

Right ventricle

FIGURE 5-5 The heart, heart valves, and an atrial septal defect.

Atheromatous plaques within the aorta in the chest can block arteries to the head. Red and white clots often form on the surface of aortic plaques. These clots as well as calcium particles and pieces of cholesterol within plaques can break loose and be carried by the bloodstream into the arteries that feed the brain.

Blood Abnormalities That Contribute to Brain Ischemia and Infarction

The ability of the blood to clot is a very important defense mechanism. Physical injuries frequently cause breakage of small blood vessels. Components of the blood plug the regions of blood vessel injury, preventing excess bleeding. A deficiency of these blood factors leads to excess bleeding; other conditions can lead to excess clotting.

The two most important parts of the body's clotting system are blood platelets and proteins within the blood and blood vessel walls that promote blood clotting. Platelets (also called thrombocytes, a term that literally means "clotting cells") are tiny cells that circulate within the blood. When there is a blood vessel injury, platelets are drawn to the injured region. They adhere to the point of injury and stick together, forming a plug. When there are too many platelets (thrombocytosis), clotting is excessive. Excess bleeding can develop when when there are too few platelets (**thrombocytopenia**). Some blood proteins (antithrombin III, protein C, and protein S) inhibit the blood from clotting when present in normal amounts. When there is a deficiency of one of these substances, usually from birth, that causes the function of other blood-clotting proteins to become excessive (e.g., factors VII, VIII, or XII), there is an increased tendency for the blood to clot. Some medical conditions (e.g., cancer) also increase clotting tendency. Acute infections and inflammatory conditions such as inflammatory bowel disease increase clotting factors and promote thrombosis. Thrombi can develop within blood vessels that have plaques and within apparently normal small blood vessels.

Conditions That Cause Brain and Subarachnoid Hemorrhage

Hypertension

Hypertension is the single most important condition that causes bleeding within the brain. Sudden increases in blood pressure severely stresses small arteries within the brain and can cause them to break with resultant hemorrhage into brain substance. Chronic, poorly controlled hypertension also wears down the walls of small arteries so that small outpouchings (micro-aneurysms) develop. These outpouchings are not visible grossly but are seen only through a microscope. The walls of these outpouchings are thin and can break especially when exposed to high blood pressure. Occasionally hypertension can cause rupture of small arteries on the surface of the brain. Bleeding in that case is subarachnoid, into the fluid around the brain. Hypertension is the single greatest risk factor for both brain infarction and brain hemorrhage. Uncontrolled hypertension was the cause of Tom M.'s cerebellar hemorrhage. His blood pressure was already high, but when he strained to lift heavy cargo, his blood pressure went even higher, causing rupture of a small artery in his left cerebellum.

Aneurysms and Vascular Malformations

Bleeding also can ensue from abnormal blood vessels. Aneurysms are outpouchings from arteries (see Figure 5-6a). They are most often located on large arteries that travel along the base of the brain. They are especially common at branch points where two arteries diverge. The walls of aneurysms are often weak in spots. These weak spots may break especially if the blood pressure is high. Rupture of aneurysms is usually into the subarachnoid space. Blood under arterial pressure suddenly enters the fluid around the brain, abruptly increasing the pressure within the head. Once an aneurysm has ruptured, there is a greatly increased likelihood that it will rupture again, often soon after the first subarachnoid bleed. Occasionally aneurysms can rupture into the brain, or more often into both the subarachnoid space and the brain. Although weak places within the artery are likely present from birth, hypertension and other factors can lead to a gradual increase in the size of aneurysms.

Vascular malformations are congenital conditions that involve blood vessels. Often also called angiomas, they usually arise from a failure of normal development of vascular networks that

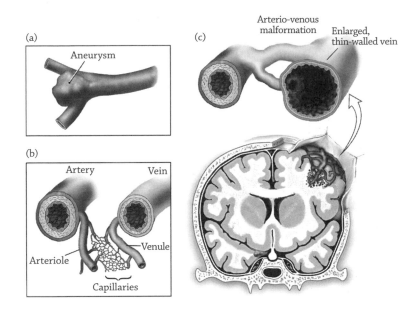

FIGURE 5-6 (a) An aneurysm located at the bifurcation of an artery.
(b) Normal communication between an artery, capillaries, and a vein.
(c) An arteriovenous malformation.

are present in the fetus before birth. Other malformations are acquired during life. There are five types of vascular malformations (see Table 5-2). Because these types are quite different, and the names and differences are complex and confusing not only to many patients who have them but also to many doctors, I will describe them in some detail.

Arteriovenous malformations (AVMs) contain arteries that communicate directly with veins. Normally blood travels from large to small arteries (arterioles) and then to a bed of tiny blood vessels called capillaries. The blood is then drained by way of the veins (see Figure 5-6b). By contrast, in an AVM blood goes directly from arteries to veins without any intervening capillary network

TABLE 5-2 Types of Vascular Malformations

Arteriovenous malformations (AVMs)
Cavernous angiomas (Cavernomas)
Developmental venous anomalies (DVAs)
Varices
Telangiectasias

(see Figure 5-6c). Veins are thin walled and are not built to withstand the pressure present in the arterial system. As a result, rupture of the veins within an AVM is common. Bleeding is usually into the brain, but can also be into the subarachnoid space if the AVM abuts the brain surface. The size of the component vessels that make up AVMs varies greatly, but the largest vessels are always veins. **Cavernous angiomas** differ from AVMs in that they have no direct arterial supply. They are composed of a relatively compact mass of tiny capillary blood vessels located close together in a capsule that separates the angioma from the rest of the brain (Figure 5-7). Most often they are located within the brain. When they bleed, the hemorrhage is usually contained within the capsule in the brain substance. Rebleeding is common and these lesions may cause seizures.

The most common type of vascular malformation found in the brain by modern brain imaging and after death were formerly called venous angiomas. Now they are more accurately called **developmental venous anomalies** (**DVAs**). In a DVA, there is a deficiency of draining veins from birth, so that those veins that do develop must drain a larger portion of brain than they are equipped to handle (Figure 5-7.) DVAs are probably not an important cause of brain hemorrhage, but they do predispose people to epileptic seizures.

Telangiectasias (very small dilated capillaries admixed with brain tissue) and **venous varices** (very dilated draining veins; see

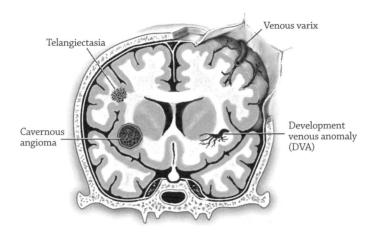

FIGURE 5-7 Cross section of the brain that contains a cavernous angioma, developmental venous anomaly, telangiectasia, and a venous varix.

Figure 5-7 for both) are the other types of vascular malformations, but they rarely cause serious brain hemorrhages.

Blood Abnormalities Can Also Promote Bleeding inside the Skull

In the Blood Abnormalities That Contribute to Brain Ischemia and Infarction section, I commented on blood components that are effective in preventing excess thrombosis. These same factors, when abnormal, can give rise to excess bleeding. A deficiency of blood platelets (thrombocytopenia) can cause hemorrhage into the skin and organs, including the brain. A deficiency of blood clotting factors can also cause hemorrhaging. The most common such situation is the prescription of anticoagulant drugs (heparin compounds, warfarin, dabigatran, apixaban, rivoraxaban). Doctors prescribe these agents to prevent clotting, but when their effects are excessive, hemorrhage can occur. In other patients, congenital deficiency of clotting factors can lead to a lifelong risk of hemorrhage. The most well-known hereditary disorder is **hemophilia,** which is a deficiency in Factor VIII (antihemophiliac globulin). Patients with bleeding tendencies usually hemorrhage into a number of different locations, but the most devastating is bleeding into the brain.

Chapter 6

Strokes and Cerebrovascular Conditions in the Young

Although strokes and damage from vascular disease are by far most common in adults and the elderly, strokes occur at all ages including, neonates, babies, young children, adolescents, and young adults. Because the underlying medical conditions and causes are different in the young, a separate chapter on this topic is warranted.

Newborns and Infants

In some children motor and other handicaps are detected after birth; these children are often classified as having **cerebral palsy**. The most common cause is loss of brain tissue due to decreased perfusion of energy-rich blood. When it became possible to image the brain and the blood vessels that supply the brain with blood, doctors found that these children had a variety of causes of decreased oxygen delivery and decreased brain perfusion during their in utero existence and delivery. Hypoxia and ischemia are most often attributable to (1) intrauterine **asphyxia**; (2) birth-related problems, such as umbilical cord prolapse, forceps delivery, or breech presentation; (3) uterine and placental abruption; (4) respiratory insufficiency after birth, caused by aspirated meconium; (5) recurrent stoppage of breathing; and (6) severe congenital heart disease. In preterm infants, fetal heart rate abnormalities, hypoglycemia, and other conditions predispose them to arterial strokes.

After delivery, brain blood flow is lower in preterm than in full-term newborns. The neonatal brain has little capability to **autoregulate** according to blood pressure and blood flow, so it is much more vulnerable to falls or elevations in blood pressure. Neonatal ischemia is often caused by cardiac disease, sepsis with vascular collapse, and hypertension. Genetic and acquired coagulation abnormalities also may contribute to the development of neonatal strokes and brain ischemia.

The most frequent resulting clinical finding is weakness, often with stiffness of the limbs (spasticity). The weakness may involve one limb (often an arm) or one side of the body: an arm and a leg, both legs, or both arms and legs. Often the muscles that control the tongue and mouth are affected so that speech is limited or slurred. Intelligence is often preserved despite the motor handicaps. Most of the damage is around the brain ventricles and the condition is referred to as **periventricular leukomalacia.**

Brain hemorrhages are an even more frequent and important cause of stroke during the perinatal period. Premature infants are especially susceptible to developing hemorrhages in the periventricular region, spreading into the ventricles. These hemorrhages start in a primitive zone deep within the brain called the subependymal germinal matrix. The matrix contains fragile capillaries and loose supporting tissue. By full term, the germinal matrix is no longer visible. Because of the lack of effective autoregulation, increases in blood pressure or blood volume can lead to breakage of these fragile vessels and resultant intracerebral hemorrhage. Most germinal matrix hemorrhages occur during the first 3 postnatal days, especially during the first postpartum hours, but some develop in utero. Clinically, infants with germinal matrix hemorrhages may appear very ill with coma, respiratory abnormalities, and poor muscle tone, or they may appear to be faring normally. At times a gradual deterioration of function occurs. Intraventricular hemorrhages can cause temporary hydrocephalus, which resolves itself, or progressive hydrocephalus, requiring ventricular drainage or shunting.

Cerebellar hemorrhage also sometimes develops during the early neonatal period, especially in premature infants.

Children and Adolescents

Brain and subarachnoid hemorrhages, injuries, infections, and congenital heart disease are important causes of stroke in children, adolescents, and young adults. In preadolescent children, vascular malformations are the most common cause of intracranial bleeding. Before age 20, subarachnoid hemorrhages due to ruptured aneurysms are a slightly more common cause of bleeding than vascular malformations.

The major causes of brain ischemia in children are (1) embolisms from the heart, (2) arterial dissections, (3) thrombosis of dural sinuses and veins, (4) **coagulopathies,** and (5) **arteriopathies.** The usual risk factors for the development of ischemic stroke in adults (hypertension, diabetes, **hyperlipidemia,** and smoking) are less important causes of brain ischemia in children.

About one-quarter of ischemic strokes in young children are attributable to heart disease. A relatively high proportion of cardiac-related ischemic strokes occur during or after surgery and other procedures. Brain infarcts in children with cardiac disease are most often caused by embolism. Bacterial endocarditis (infection of valves in the heart) is an important cause. Congenital heart disease, especially with shunting of blood (atrial and ventricular septal defects including patent foramen ovale [PFO] and patent ductus arteriosis) and complex congenital defects, are frequent. Children with stroke and congenital heart disease are often cyanotic and have chronic hypoxia and increased red blood cell counts (**polycythemia**). They may develop venous and arterial occlusions as a result of the polycythemia. Rheumatic heart disease, endocarditis, cardiomyopathies, and myocarditis are important acquired heart diseases associated with brain embolism.

Arterial composition and function in childhood is different from that in most adults, since the intracranial arteries are
rarely subject to important degenerative atherosclerotic changes.
Increased vascular elasticity and reactivity contribute to the development of so-called **arteriopathy** in this age group from a variety
of different stimuli. Arteriopathies are characterized by local and
generalized regions of narrowing, occlusion, or dilation of intracranial large arteries. Arteriopathies have a variety of different
causes including infection, trauma, migraine, moyamoya disease,
and genetic conditions such as sickle-cell disease, **Fabry disease**,
and **mitochondrial disorders**. The presence of an angiographi-
cally confirmed arteriopathy conveys an increased risk for stroke
recurrence.

Moyamoya disease is a condition of unknown cause that develops in children and young adults in which the carotid arteries within
the skull become gradually occluded. As the vessels occlude, many
small, deep blood vessels enlarge. The vessels resemble a puff of
smoke—the English translation of the Japanese term *moyamoya*.
These abnormalities can lead to brain infarction or hemorrhage.

One important cause of arteriopathy in childhood is trauma.
Direct trauma can lead to arterial occlusion and intense vasoconstriction. Stretching of arteries at locations where they are not
anchored can lead to tearing of arterial walls (dissections). Head and
neck traumas, even trivial ones, are often mentioned as a predispos-
ing factor by the parents of children with ischemic strokes. Young
children may fall while keeping pencils and toothbrushes in their
mouths, injuring or lacerating the pharynx and the internal carotid
artery during its course behind the tonsillar pillars in the throat.
Carotid and vertebral artery dissections in the neck can develop
after head or neck injuries, especially involving sudden twisting
movements and blunt trauma to the neck. Neck, jaw, or throat pain
or headache may be the earliest symptoms. Brain infarction occurs
when the blood within the arterial wall dissects into the arterial
lumen and embolizes intracranially. At times, the intramural clot

occludes the lumen sufficiently that a luminal thrombus forms because of sluggish flow and activation of clotting factors. Even trivial head trauma is occasionally the cause of severe intracranial arterial dissections.

Infections can directly cause or predispose to strokes in children. Tonsillitis can occasionally lead to occlusive changes in the adjacent pharyngeal portion of the internal carotid artery. Influenza, *Mycoplasma pneumoniae,* and enterovirus infections have occasionally been implicated as causes of brain infarction. HIV (the cause of AIDS) and the spirochetes that cause Lyme disease and syphilis are other known causes of arteriopathy. The best studied infectious cause of arteriopathy is infection with the varicella zoster virus (VZV) that causes chicken pox and shingles (herpes zoster). This virus has an affinity for nerves and blood vessels. Particles characteristic of VZV can be found in the nuclei and cytoplasm of smooth-muscle cells in involved arteries. VZV gains access to brain arteries by way of the **meninges** and through nerves that innervate the arteries. Endothelial viral infection could cause thrombosis by activating platelets and triggering coagulation. Endothelial perturbation could lead to vasoconstriction, compromising the delivery of blood and presenting as an arteriopathy.

Post-varicella arteriopathy and brain infarction have now been studied extensively in children. In one large study of children with chicken pox, children acquired a varicella infection at 1 to 10.4 years of age (median = 4.4 years) and had their first episode of brain ischemia 4 to 47 weeks later (median = 17 weeks). Brain ischemic episodes recurred, either acutely or during the 1 to 33 weeks after symptom onset, often associated with progression of abnormalities on vascular imaging. Angiograms showed single regions of focal ringlike stenosis and gradual longer segments of stenosis and multifocal narrowings. In some patients stenosis was maximal on initial studies, but often later progressed to involve previously uninvolved arteries. The vascular abnormalities improved or completely regressed during follow-up over 6 to 79 months.

Migraine is also common in children with brain infarcts. Migraine probably causes brain infarcts by prolonged vasoconstriction or the formation of local thrombi related to vascular narrowing and activation of the clotting system. Children's blood vessels are more prone to vasoconstriction then in adulthood.

Young Adults (20–40 Years)

Atherosclerosis is a much less common cause of stroke in young adults than in the older age groups. However, severe hypertension, insulin-dependent diabetes, smoking, and very high lipid levels can lead to premature atherosclerosis and strokes among young adults.

In Table 6-1 I list the conditions that are more frequent in individuals under 40 than in the older age groups. Arterial dissections occur more often in young adults probably because of more frequent athletic activities and vigorous exercise and the mobility of youthful nonsclerotic arteries. Mobile arteries are more readily torn during sudden or extreme head and neck movements and with trauma. Claire H. developed a carotid artery dissection during sports activities. If strokes such as paradoxical embolism are to occur from congenital lesions (e.g., PFOs), they will most often do so before middle age. By late adulthood, some PFOs close and other stroke causes predominate. Other congenital vascular lesions that cause bleeding (aneurysms, AVMs, and cavernomas) often present during the twenties and thirties. Unfortunately, illicit drug use, a plague among adolescents and young adults, continues to be a frequent cause of strokes. Amphetamines cause mostly brain hemorrhages, while cocaine can cause both hemorrhagic and ischemic strokes. Heroin and drugs packaged for oral use but injected intravenously can cause brain infarcts.

There is a small increase in the risk of stroke during pregnancy and the puerperium (the weeks after delivery) and when taking pills containing female hormones. Eclampsia, severe vasoconstriction,

TABLE 6-1 Important Causes of Stroke in Young Adults

1. Arterial dissections
2. Paradoxical embolism (PFO)
3. Hemorrhages: aneurysms, AVMs, cavernomas
4. Illicit drugs: amphetamines, cocaine, heroin
5. Venous sinus thrombosis
6. Pregnancy and puerperium related: eclampsia, RCVS, venous thrombosis
7. Systemic illness and infection related
   Cancer
   Leukemia
   Bacterial endocarditis
   HIV/AIDS
   Tuberculosis
   Cysticercosis
   Syphilis
   Crohn's disease, ulcerative colitis, rheumatoid arthritis
   Systemic lupus erythematosis

PFO = patent foramen ovale; AVM = arteriovenous malformation;
RCVS = reversible cerebral vasoconstriction syndrome; HIV/AIDS = human
immunodeficiency virus/acquired immunodeficiency syndrome.

and thrombosis of veins inside the cranium are the most frequent causes of stroke in these women. Heart disease and other conditions present before pregnancy can also promote strokes during pregnancy and the puerperium.

In many young adults, strokes are directly related to systemic conditions and infections. Cancer and leukemia affect blood clotting and can cause both ischemic and hemorrhagic strokes. Some infections directly or indirectly affect the blood vessels inside the head. Tuberculosis, syphilis, and cysticercosis (the disease related to ingestion of the eggs of the pork tapeworm) are examples of infections that can cause brain ischemia. Bacterial endocarditis is an infection of the heart valves that causes strokes via embolization of the infectious material that creates a vegetation on the surface of the valves. In patients with HIV/AIDS, enhanced clotting can develop and superimposed infections can directly affect brain blood vessels. Inflammatory conditions such as Crohn's disease, ulcerative colitis, and rheumatoid arthritis can cause enhanced clotting and lead to thrombosis of arteries and veins in the head. Systemic lupus erythematosus, a condition that is most prevalent in young women, leads to strokes by causing heart valve lesions and blood abnormalities.

Because strokes and cerebrovascular abnormalities have so many potential causes in children and young adults, the evaluation and tests are often more extensive and diverse than in the elderly.

Chapter 7

What Are the Different Symptoms of Stroke? What Abnormalities Do Doctors Look for and Find in Stroke Patients?

Good medical care involves full cooperation and interaction between patients and doctors. Of course doctors cannot treat individuals unless they first come to them with their symptoms. Symptoms develop when individuals become aware of changes in any of the usual functions of their bodies. Since brain tissue is so vulnerable to changes in its blood supply, the timing of treatment can be critical. The adage "time = brain" was coined to emphasize the importance of rapid treatment of any circulatory problem that threatens to injure the brain. In order to present to doctors quickly, individuals must become aware of what symptoms suggest that a person is having or might develop a stroke.

Many surveys and reports show that the general public is woefully ignorant and unaware of the symptoms and causes of stroke. A recent survey was given in the UK to 622 individuals who had had strokes in the past (Slark J, Bentley P, Majeed A, Sharma P. Awareness of Stroke Symptomatology and Cardiovascular Risk Factors amongst Stroke Survivors. *J Stroke and Cerebrovasc Dis* 2012;21:358–362). When asked what were the three most common stroke symptoms, only one in seven named all three (face and/or arm weakness, leg weakness, speech disturbance) and a third knew none of the three. They were also generally unaware of the major risk factors for stroke. Sadly, they also failed to recognize that their own major risk factors had contributed to their having had a stroke and posed risks for another stroke. If stroke survivors who presumably were given information about stroke and their own risks failed these questions, imagine what the responses would be among individuals in the general public who were naïve to stroke. Because of this naïveté, I chose to discuss the brain and its functions in the first chapters, since that information is most relevant to understanding stroke symptoms.

There are two different types of symptoms: those that reflect loss of function of parts of the brain, and those that relate to the vascular cause of the brain injury. Lets illustrate the two types of symptoms by referring to Elaine S., a woman I first mentioned in the Chapter 1:

> Recall that Elaine S was an 82-year-old woman. Her health had always been good. Recently she noticed episodes when her heart beat fast and irregularly. This would last from 2 to 15 minutes and worried her, but she did not tell her doctor. One afternoon she suddenly realized that her left hand and leg had become weak and she felt tingling over the entire left side of her body, including her face. When she was examined at the hospital, doctors noted that she had atrial fibrillation. Her left atrium was not contracting normally enough to efficiently eject blood into the left ventricle. A clot had formed in the enlarged and inefficiently contracting left atrium, which then embolized to a blood vessel supplying the right side of the brain, causing infarction.

In this example, the bouts of rapid irregular heartbeat were symptoms of atrial fibrillation. I discussed this heart condition in Chapter 5, which lists medical conditions that cause strokes. The left limb weakness and the numbness of the left side of the body developed because of loss of function of regions within the right cerebral hemisphere of the brain. In very simple terms, the symptoms caused by atrial fibrillation gave a clue to *what* was wrong, and the nature of the brain symptoms gave information that the brain was involved and about *where* the problem was in the brain.

Both the *what* and *where* questions are important. For Elaine S., the doctor's examination allowed her to recognize that the brain problem was located within the region near the central sulcus within the right cerebral hemisphere. (Refer to Chapter 2, which describes this area.) An image of the brain, such as a CT or MRI scan, might show the regions involved and corroborate the doctor's clinical impression. Her physician knew that the right middle cerebral artery branch of the right internal carotid artery supplied this region. Something must have happened to this arterial pathway. This anatomical information (discussed in Chapter 3) could lead the doctor to obtain images of these involved blood vessels and the heart. Clearly, identifying the *what* aspect, atrial fibrillation, allows the physician to emphasize heart evaluation and embolism from the heart as an important cause of the stroke.

In this chapter I will discuss the symptoms caused by abnormal brain function (the *where* question), and the symptoms that relate to the medical condition that cause stroke (the *what* question), separately. I must first warn readers that neither the brain symptoms nor the medical condition symptoms are specific for stroke. Loss of brain functions can be caused by many different conditions, not just stroke. Also, neurologic symptoms can come from parts of the nervous system other than the brain. Everyone has had the experience of having their hand or leg go numb when nerves in that limb have been compressed; for example, by sitting with the legs crossed for some time. The timing of when and how the symptoms developed and changed is often more important in diagnosing stroke as compared to other conditions. Strokes usually come on suddenly. A person who has a stroke literally is abruptly *stricken* with brain symptoms. Only a very small minority of strokes develop gradually. Similarly, symptoms that accompany medical conditions, such as headache, vomiting, neck discomfort, and chest pain, can also be nonspecific.

Symptoms Due to Loss of Brain Function

I hope that the discussion in Chapter 2 of what the brain looks like and how it works will help readers anticipate what symptoms might develop when parts of the brain stop functioning normally, and where in the brain those functions might be located. Please refer back to that chapter as I discuss the common neurologic stroke-related symptoms.

Weakness

Loss of strength and coordination in one or more limbs is a common stroke symptom. In fact, most people equate stroke with paralysis. Although weakness is a very common symptom, many strokes do not cause it. Weakness is noted when someone uses a limb and finds that it does not have normal power. By contrast, numbness can be recognized at rest as a lack of feeling in a body part without having to use it. Individuals often confuse the two symptoms. Weakness can involve one body part (e.g., a hand), but more often weakness involves more than one area on the same side of the body. The severity of the loss of power can vary from slight to total inability to move a body part: paralysis. Elaine S. noticed weakness in her left arm and leg. Claire H. developed weakness in her right arm and hand. Face, arm, and hand; arm and leg; and face, arm, and leg are common locations for weakness to develop in stroke patients. Occasionally when a critical blood vessel that supplies the brainstem is involved, both sides of the body and all four limbs can become weak at the same time.

Loss of strength is usually due to involvement of the motor region in the gyrus, just before the central sulcus, in the cerebral hemisphere opposite to the side of the weakness or to the pathway (pyramidal tract) that passes through the cerebral hemispheres and the brainstem.

Numbness

Different individuals use the word *numb* to mean quite different things. The commonest usage is a loss of the ability to feel in the numb areas. Some speak of a loss of sensation as if the area had been injected with novocaine. "Prickling," "tingling," and "falling asleep" are other words patients often use. Occasionally the sensations described are unpleasant: burning, hot, oversensitive to touch, or an unpleasant feeling when warm or cold objects are placed on the numb area. The numbness can involve just one limb or part of a limb, or, like weakness, it can involve multiple regions on one side of the body. Sometimes the numbness involves the face, arm, leg, and trunk on one side of the body as it did in Elaine S. Some patients describe the distribution as if a line was drawn right down the midline of their body, with everything on one side of the line becoming numb. Often numbness and weakness are described together in the limbs or face on one side of the body. Robert H. had spells when his left hand and arm felt numb. When his stroke developed, his whole left side went numb as well as weak.

The sensory zones in the cerebral hemispheres lie just behind the motor zones in the gyrus, behind the central sulcus in the hemisphere opposite to the side that is numb, or in the pathways in the brainstem and cerebral hemispheres that convey the information to the sensory cortex in the cerebral hemispheres. The lateral portion of the thalamus is an important way station for incoming sensory stimuli; it is involved in many patients in whom numbness involves one-half of the body.

Disturbances of Vision

Visual loss is another common symptom present during strokes and TIAs. The brain contains a wide range of structures that relate to seeing and looking. Chapter 2 discusses the pathways from the eye to the cerebral cortex in the occipital lobes that are specialized for interpretation of visual information.

Visual loss can involve one eye (dubbed **monocular visual loss**). The first branch of the internal carotid artery is the ophthalmic artery, the main blood supply of the eye. When the carotid artery is narrowed, patients often develop temporary visual loss in the eye. They often describe a shade coming down from the top and gradually blocking vision in that eye. For others, the shade comes across the eye like a curtain being pulled from the side. Sometimes the vision in one eye just becomes grey or black. In situations in which the blood pressure becomes very low, visual loss can occur at the same time in both eyes.

Interruption of blood supply often involves one or both posterior cerebral arteries, vessels that supply the regions on each side of the brain that receive visual messages from objects on the opposite side of the environment. (See the description of these arteries in Chapter 3.) Blockage of the right posterior cerebral artery causes patients to become unable to see well toward their left, and blockage of the left posterior cerebral artery impairs vision to the right. Some patients do not recognize the loss of their span of vision and only become aware that something is wrong when they collide with objects or cars on their blind side. At times patients become aware of "holes" in their vision on one side. In rare cases, an embolus that blocks both posterior cerebral arteries causes patients to become effectively blind.

Less common are visual illusions and distortion of objects. Some brain lesions cause objects to seem tilted, or abnormally small or large. Some patients lose the ability to perceive the color of objects, or can no longer judge distances or detect movement of objects in one part of their field of vision.

Double vision (diplopia) is another common symptom. It is caused by the two eyes not working together normally. The two objects can be horizontally, vertically, or obliquely displaced. Often the objects become further apart when the patient looks to one side or up and down. The cause most often relates either to involvement of one of the nerves that supplies a muscle that moves the eyes, or to a stroke in the brainstem where the nerve cells that control the eye muscles are located. Abnormal perception of movement and oscillation of objects are discussed in the next section.

Dizziness, Vertigo, and Loss of Balance and Coordination

Structures in the inner ear and in the brainstem and cerebellum help us maintain our balance and equilibrium. When these structures are impaired, individuals report dizziness. Sometimes they describe frank **vertigo**, a sensation that they or the room is moving or turning. Double vision and the sensation that objects are oscillating are other descriptions they mention.

The abnormality can occur primarily when walking. Individuals may veer or lean to one side, or stagger from one side to another. Tom M. had dizziness and severe loss of balance when a hemorrhage developed in his cerebellum. In some cases, just the limbs on one side become uncoordinated or shake (tremor) when an individual attempts to grab an object with his or her hand.

The brainstem regions that receive information from the ear structures relating to balance are called vestibular nuclei. They are located in the tegmentum of the medulla and lower pons, and are interrelated to areas in the middle of the cerebellum that relate to balance and walking and coordinating the arms and legs.

Speech and Language

Two different types of speaking abnormalities can be symptoms of stroke: dysarthria and aphasia. In **dysarthria**, stroke patients have difficulty pronouncing words. This abnormality is related to weakness of the muscles that are used in talking: those in the face, mouth, lips, tongue, pharynx, and jaw. Dysarthric patients may be difficult to understand because they slur words, but the words that they do say are correct, and they understand speech and write language normally (if their hand is not too weak to write).

Aphasia, in contrast to dysarthria, is an abnormality of language. Stroke patients may use wrong words, and the phrases that they speak may not be linguistically or grammatically correct. Some aphasics also have difficulty understanding the meaning of either spoken or written language. The language abnormalities may include reading, writing, and spelling.

Language abnormalities in nearly all right-handed and four-fifths of left-handed individuals are caused by strokes in the left cerebral hemisphere, in areas surrounding the sylvian fissure that are devoted to language. Dysarthria can be caused by an abnormality of any brain region that causes weakness or incoordination of the muscles used in talking. Weakness of the face and or limbs on one side of the body is usually but not always present. Since the same muscles are used in swallowing, many patients with dysarthria also have **dysphagia**—difficulty in swallowing.

Abnormalities of Memory, Thinking, and Behavior

A large part of the human brain is concerned with thinking, memory, interpreting visual space, and governing how a person acts. Abnormalities of these functions are common in stroke patients, but they are most often accompanied by abnormalities already discussed: weakness, numbness, visual loss, abnormal walking and coordination, and abnormal speech.

Some stroke patients develop difficulty retaining and remembering events and discussions. Memory loss in these patients develops suddenly. They tend to repeat stories and questions, and don't recall answers or things that have happened recently. The abnormality is most often localized to the hippocampal structures in the medial temporal lobes, or in structures that connect to the hippocampi.

Some stroke patients seem not to be aware of objects or people on one side of their environment. They often ignore things and people on their left side. This abnormality is referred to as neglect of one side of space. Other patients lose their sense of space and proportions. They cannot recall where things are located and cannot draw or even copy visually simple objects. They may get lost in areas that were formerly familiar to them—even their own home. These visual-spatial abnormalities are often present in patients who have stroke damage in the right cerebral hemisphere. Patients with large strokes in this region may be completely unaware of having any deficit; they may even fail to recognize or acknowledge that they cannot use their left limbs.

In some patients the change in function relates to the quantity of their behavior and interactions. They may do much less and be content to sit without much spontaneous action or speech. They lose interest in activities, reading, hobbies, and other people. Their families and friends may say that they have become "couch potatoes" or say that they act like "a bump on a log." Other patients may become very restless and hyperactive. They may talk incessantly, much more than usual. One topic may merge into another. These individuals appear agitated, restless, and hyperactive. These abnormalities often are explained by strokes that involve the caudate nuclei, the thalamus, or the frontal or temporal lobes of the cerebral hemispheres.

Sleepiness, Lethargy, Stupor, and Coma

These terms all refer to a decrease in the level of consciousness. In some patients with stroke, decreased alertness and loss of consciousness are the predominant features. Usually this means that the stroke is serious. Either a large portion of brain is involved, or pressure inside the head is increased, or the regions in the brainstem that control consciousness have been affected. Bleeding into the brain or the subarachnoid space is a common cause.

Summing up the Symptoms to Locate the Part of the Brain Involved

Doctors consider all of the symptoms when trying to discover where in the brain the dysfunction lies. For example, Elaine S., the patient described at the beginning of this chapter, had symptoms of weakness in her left hand and leg, and loss of sensation involving the left limbs and side of the body. The abnormality in the brain either would have to involve the precentral motor cortex and the adjacent postcentral gyrus sensory regions toward the top of the brain, or interrupt the pathways from those regions. If the abnormality included the parietal lobe behind the postcentral gyrus, then a disability of drawing and copying things, and some neglect of objects to the left, might also be found on examination. The general principle that doctors use for stroke location is to develop a hypothesis of what structures are involved. They then can test for abnormalities that could localize the abnormality more precisely.

Robert H. suddenly developed left limb paralysis, along with neglect of the left side of visual space, and was completely unaware of his loss of function. These symptoms indicate a large abnormality in the right cerebral hemisphere. Claire H.'s speech disability and right limb paralysis pointed to a left cerebral problem involving the speech region. In Tom M.'s case, his loss of balance when walking, lurching to the left, and dizziness suggested an abnormality in the left side of the cerebellum.

Symptoms That Relate to Stroke Cause

Few symptoms are specific for stroke or for the different subtypes of stroke. For Elaine S., the irregular heartbeat strongly suggested a heart rhythm disturbance and that the stroke was due to embolism from the heart. In some patients, headache precedes or accompanies the stroke. Headache can result from blockage of blood vessels and dilation of other blood vessels to take up the slack. Headache can also result from high blood pressure. Tom M. had headache, vomiting, and decreased consciousness at the onset of his stroke—a hypertensive brain hemorrhage.

What Findings Do Doctors Look for in Patients Suspected of Having a Stroke?

Physical findings and symptoms are divided into those that relate to brain dysfunction and those that relate to the vascular cause. Heart and vascular examinations seek abnormalities that might be stroke related. Doctors check the pulse at the wrist to determine the heart rate and regularity. They also check blood pressure and listen to the heart. They listen for murmurs that might suggest abnormalities of the heart valves and heart contractions. They may check the carotid, subclavian, and innominate artery pulses in the neck. Often they will listen to the neck arteries and even to the eyes. They are listening for bruits, a French term for noise that is audible along the arteries, which suggests that the artery might be narrowed at the point the bruit is heard. Doctors may also examine the abdomen and feel the pulses in the feet.

Neurologic testing varies with the type of symptoms and the time available for the examination. I will describe a relatively complete examination, but every doctor might not perform a complete examination on every patient. To convey the parts of the examination, it is easiest for me to describe what I usually do. I am seeking the abnormalities of brain function described earlier under the categories of symptoms. The examination is described here to familiarize you with what your doctor may do to determine if there are functional abnormalities of any part of your nervous system.

The conversation in which patients describe symptoms and events and respond to my questions tells me about their speech, pronunciation, and ability to understand spoken language. To test speech further I often ask patients to repeat phrases and to name objects that I point to in the room and in my doctor bag. I ask them to read a paragraph and to write a brief paragraph about the city in which they live or another familiar topic. I usually show pictures of several scenes that I carry in my bag and ask patients to describe them after I have removed the scene from view. This tells me something about their visual-spatial abilities, their thoroughness in scanning the full scene and recognizing details, and the language that they use in telling me what they see. To test these functions further, I also ask patients to draw a clock, bicycle, daisy, or another familiar object from memory, and then to copy a complex diagram that I draw. I then often show them photographs of seven to 10 famous individuals (presidents, sports figures, entertainers, etc.), asking them to describe and name these people. To test memory, I then ask patients to try and recall the paragraph that they read, the scenes that they saw, and the individual photographs that I showed them.

I then begin to test the functions of the structures in the face and head. I test visual acuity in each eye with a handheld eye chart. I then ask patients to face me as I bring my fingers or an object into their vision from each side to determine if peripheral vision has been preserved. I then look with an **ophthalmoscope** at the blood vessels and nerves within the eyes. I then look at the pupil and lids of each eye, and test the movements of each eye and of the eyes moving together to each side and up and down. I then test movements of the face, throat, and tongue, and hearing in each ear. Feeling on the face is tested with cotton, touch, and a cold object.

Moving down to the arms, I see if the arms are of equal strength by asking patients to hold their arms out in front of them to see if one side drifts downward, indicating weakness. I test the muscles of the arms at the shoulders, elbow, wrist, and hand on both sides in turn. Then with a reflex hammer I test the reflexes at the elbows and wrists, and test feeling in the arms using cotton, touch, and sometimes a pin. I move the fingers slightly up or down while the patients' eyes are closed to see if they can detect the direction of movement. I also see if they can feel the vibrations of a tuning fork placed on their fingers.

I then move to the lower limbs and test them in the same way I tested the upper limbs, analyzing strength, reflexes, and feeling. Watching patients stand and walk is another very important part of the examination. I usually watch their gait as they proceed into the examination room, or at the very end of the examination if they were first met and examined in their room in a hospital bed.

When Claire H. was examined, she was alert but used wrong or nonexistent words. She could not read. Her visual functions were normal. Her right hand was weak but her right leg had normal strength, and she could feel touch, cold, and the vibrations of a tuning fork normally on both her right and left hands, feet, and body. These findings made it clear that her problem could only be localized to the left cerebral hemisphere, in a region above and below the sylvian fissure, in areas that relate to language function.

Examination of Robert H. showed complete paralysis of his left arm, hand, and leg. He could not appreciate or localize touch or cold objects placed on his left side. He could not see to his left. Despite these abnormalities, when asked, he did not think anything was wrong with him. He clearly had sustained severe damage to a large area on the right side of the brain.

By the time Elaine S. was examined, her left limbs had improved and were only slightly weak. She had difficulty feeling a soft cotton touch on her left hand and foot, and she could not appreciate fine movements of her left fingers. Cold objects felt less cold on her left arm, hand, and leg. Her reflexes were brisker on the left than the same areas on the right. These abnormalities localized to the right parietal lobe region of her brain. Some of her symptoms had improved, so that she was better than she had been when she first developed the neurologic symptoms. When her symptoms first developed, she likely had a larger area of lower blood flow located in front of the central sulcus that improved when her embolus moved along.

When Tom M. attempted to sit or stand, he leaned to the left. He could not walk. When he attempted to walk, he lurched in a drunken fashion to his left side. His left arm and hand were quite clumsy when he attempted to reach for an object. These findings reinforced the idea that his left cerebellum was not functioning normally.

Having determined the nature of the patient's symptoms, and the abnormalities found on examination, the doctor is in a position to order images and laboratory tests to better pinpoint any abnormalities in the brain and blood, the heart, and the blood vessels that supply the brain. I will discuss these tests in Chapter 9 after first discussing risk factors for stroke.

Chapter 8

What Are the Risk Factors for Stroke and How Can They Be Reduced?

Strokes do not just develop "out of the blue." Most often there are **risk factors** and behaviors that predispose individuals to develop a stroke. Genetics also plays an important role. In this chapter I introduce and discuss these risk factors to familiarize readers with their management.

Transient Ischemic Attacks

The most important alarm requiring immediate, rapid attention is an attack in which a person temporarily loses normal function of a part of the brain. The vascular problems that cause strokes often cause temporary symptoms. When these spells are caused by an abnormality of the blood supply to the brain, they are referred to as transient ischemic attacks (TIAs) or sometimes "brain attacks." The symptoms in these attacks are the same as those that occur during a stroke, except that they are temporary, often lasting only a few minutes, most often less than an hour. The most frequent symptoms are listed in Table 8-1.

A TIA signals trouble in the arteries that bring oxygen, sugar, and other nutrients necessary for survival of brain tissue. When the lack of blood flow is brief or relatively minor, temporary loss of function develops but resolves when blood flow is restored. TIAs are caused by temporary blockage of an artery by a passing blood clot or a temporary inadequacy of blood flow through a narrowed artery.

TABLE 8-1 Common Symptoms during TIAs

Weakness of an arm or leg, or both the arm and the leg on one side of the body
Numbness of the face; arm or leg; or face, arm and leg on one side
Temporary loss of vision in one eye
Double vision
Loss of the ability to speak normally
Incoordination of the limbs or imbalance when walking
Dizziness and loss of balance

These brief attacks indicate that something is wrong with the system and so warn of the possibility of a stroke. The risk of developing a stroke is highest in the hours, days, and weeks after a TIA. Since no one can predict when a stroke might occur, immediate medical care is strongly recommended. Finding the abnormality causing the symptoms and fixing it can prevent a stroke. Studies show that outcomes are greatly improved when individuals who have had a TIA are evaluated soon after the attack by individuals with training and experience in cerebrovascular disease.

Robert H., the first patient introduced in Chapter 1, had several TIAs before his stroke. The first attack lasted 15 minutes and involved numbness and weakness of his left hand and arm. He assumed that he had leaned on the hand for too long. Two days later, shortly after he awakened in the morning, his left face and hand became numb and tingly for about 5 minutes. That same day, he had a brief attack of decreased vision in the right eye that lasted only a minute or so. He did not understand the significance of his symptoms and scheduled a routine appointment with his family physician and an eye doctor. Before he saw these doctors he had a major stroke. If he had been evaluated quickly, carotid artery disease, the cause of his symptoms, would have been detected and treated and his stroke most likely would have been prevented.

When doctors recognize that the symptoms indicate TIAs, they can often diagnose the medical abnormality and give treatments that can prevent a stroke from developing. Individuals who have a TIA should seek care in medical centers that have the doctors and technology to determine their particular problem quickly. Neurologists are especially trained to diagnose and care for stroke patients. Also, some hospitals have been designated Primary and Comprehensive Stroke Centers. These centers have shown that they are capable of effectively diagnosing and treating patients with cerebrovascular disease. It is important to know where these centers are in the area where you live.

Early Knowledge of Risk Factors Is the Key to Prevention

The key words related to prevention of stroke are *individual stroke risk factors*. Chapters 4, 5 and 6 should have made it clear to readers that strokes can be caused by many different conditions. Each individual should become aware of their own risks and behaviors that might predispose them to have a stroke, and at a relatively early age. Prevention should begin early in life and continue throughout life. There is much that everyone can and should do to prevent stroke.

Some risk factors are beyond control. For instance, we know that age, male sex, and a history of stroke in close family members are risk factors for stroke. As you get older, you have a greater chance of having a stroke. If you are male, your chances of stroke before age 60 are higher than if you are female. If a parent or sibling has coronary heart disease or stroke, you have a higher chance of stroke than a person whose family members do not have a history of vascular disease. But of course you cannot choose your parents or your sex, and living long enough to become old is a goal that everyone shares.

Unfortunately, many individuals think of risk factors and prevention only after they have had a stroke or heart attack. Prevention after an event is called secondary prevention. Thinking about prevention after an event like a bad stroke or a severe heart attack is like shutting the barn door after the horse is already out of the barn. Primary prevention—that is, prevention before a condition occurs—is much preferred. We now know that most medical risk factors and situations that increase stroke risk begin rather early in life. When teenagers and young people in their twenties die after accidents, their blood vessels often show early indications of atherosclerosis, a degenerative condition that leads to heart attacks and strokes and that increases with time.

Years ago I heard a presentation from an Alabama school teacher that brought home to me the message that risk factors develop rather early in life. This teacher asked her sixth-grade students about medical conditions that had occurred in their own families. Most of the children had very little information about their families' medical problems. After all, many parents don't want to frighten their children with information about their own medical problems and history. The teacher then gave the children a homework assignment: go home and ask your father and mother, and any older brothers and sisters, about their medical conditions, and about any illnesses and conditions among grandparents and other close relatives such as aunts and uncles, and bring this information to class. The teacher asked a pediatrician to examine the children after their families' medical conditions had been recorded.

The assignment revealed that when parents had a history of high blood pressure, their sons and daughters often also had blood pressures that were higher than average for their age. When the family history included diabetes, the students often had higher than normal blood sugar. When mom or dad was obese, their children were often heavy. This experiment shows how risk factors for vascular disease are often present very early in life and should be addressed early—before the damage occurs.

Risk factors can be divided into those that are medical and those that relate to a variety of different activities, lifestyles, and behaviors. It is to be hoped that many individuals will be able to modify behaviors found to be risk factors for stroke. Many of the medical conditions also can be prevented or minimized by behavior change and medical treatments. Figure 8-1 shows the attributable risks of 10 of the risk factors that account for 90 percent of ischemic strokes.

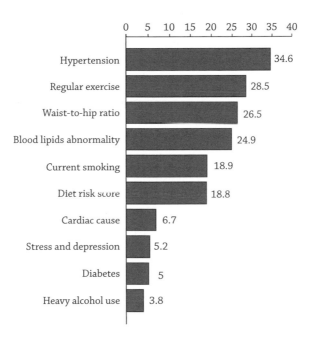

FIGURE 8-1 Source: Based on data from Testai F, Gorelick PB. Potential for stroke prevention. In: Spence D, Barnett HJM. eds. *Stroke Prevention.* New York: McGraw-Hill; 2012:22–38.

Medical Risk Factors

Hypertension

High blood pressure (hypertension) is the single most important modifiable risk factor for stroke. It is associated with a two- to three-fold increase in the risk of stroke and accounts for almost a third of stroke risk. High blood pressure is very common; many individuals over 60 have higher than normal blood pressure. Hypertension is especially common among African Americans and Asians, and it often runs in families.

Elevated blood pressure causes wear and tear on blood vessels that supply the brain with blood. To use our earlier plumbing analogy, if the pipes in a home had water that flowed under higher than normal pressure, they would become damaged sooner than if water pressures were low. When pressure becomes very high, pipes can become thin in places and leak. Similarly, when blood pressure is very high, blood vessels can break, leading to bleeding around and in the brain. Chronic high blood pressure causes thickening of arteries and leads to atherosclerosis and narrowing of arteries, which can deprive the brain of needed blood flow. Robert H. had a family history of hypertension, and he himself had had high blood pressure for 20 years before his stroke. The stroke was caused by development of severe carotid artery atherosclerosis, undoubtedly related to Robert's hypertension. Tom M. had been told that his blood pressure was high, but he ignored this warning and eventually developed a brain hemorrhage related to uncontrolled high blood pressure.

Every study of high blood pressure has shown that it is under-recognized and undertreated. One study of 50 million Americans found that just under a third of patients (16 million) had high blood pressure but did not know it. Another 15 percent (7.5 million) of individuals had hypertension but were receiving no treatment. About a quarter (13 million) were being treated, but their blood pressures were not well controlled. Only 27 percent (13.5 million) of these individuals had hypertension that was being well controlled by treatment.

Blood pressure should be checked even in young people. In individuals who have elevated blood pressures, home measurement of blood pressures using easily available measuring devices is important. Unfortunately, measurement of blood pressure in doctor's offices every few months does not give a true picture of the everyday level of blood pressure. So-called white coat hypertension is common. This term refers to the fact that patients often become nervous when seeing a doctor, and their blood pressure rises. However, these same individuals often have elevated blood pressure when confronted with stressful situations in their everyday lives. Multiple measurement of blood pressure in different circumstances and at different times of the day gives treating doctors a truer pattern of blood pressure than casual, infrequent measurement in doctors' offices. Blood pressure measuring devices are readily available and are not expensive. Doctors also can order a monitoring device that records blood pressure throughout the day and at night. This gives them the information they need to prescribe the best treatments for getting blood pressure to normal levels and keeping them there.

Changes in activity level and diet can reduce elevated blood pressure. In overweight individuals, weight loss can reduce blood pressure substantially. Regular physical exercise, decreasing alcohol intake, and reducing salt in the diet are also useful blood-pressure-reducing measures. Do not add salt to food or while cooking, and check nutrition labels for the word *sodium* in such ingredients as sodium chloride (table salt), sodium alginate, sodium benzoate, sodium bicarbonate (baking soda), monosodium glutamate (MSG), and so forth. Instead of table salt, use pepper, fresh herbs, or citrus zest to add flavor. Birth control pills can elevate blood pressure substantially in some women; stopping these pills will normalize blood pressure.

Table 8-2 lists various classes of drugs, and the most common drugs within each class that doctors prescribe to lower blood pressure. Medicines to control hypertension have proliferated over recent decades, so treatment for each individual has to be tailored and monitored to determine its effectiveness. Strategies that lower blood pressure in one patient may not work in others.

TABLE 8-2 Drugs Used to Treat Hypertension, Organized by Class

Diuretics
    Hydrochlorothiazide
    Chlorthalidone
    Indapamide
    Furosemide
    Ethacrynic acid
    Triamterene
    Amiloride
Aldosterone antagonists
    Spironolactone
    Eplerenone
Adrenergic agents
    Beta-blockers
        Propranolol
        Atenolol
        Metoprolol
        Nadolol
        Bisoprolol
        Pindolol
        Timolol
    Alpha-blockers
        Doxazosin
        Terazosin
        Prazosin
    Combined alpha- and beta-blockers
        Labetalol
        Carvedilol

TABLE 8-2 (Continued)

Centrally acting adrenergic inhibitors
  Clonidine
  Methyldopa
Peripherally active adrenergic inhibitors (seldom now used)
  Reserpine
  Guanethidine
Calcium channel blockers
  Verapamil
  Amlodipine
  Nicardipine
  Nifedipine
  Diltiazem
  Felodipine
Angiotensin converting enzyme (ACE) inhibitors
  Perindopril
  Lisinopril
  Captopril
  Enalapril
  Ramipril
  Trandolapril
  Quinapril
  Moexipril
  Benazepril
Angiotensin receptor blockers (ARBs)
  Losartan
  Valsartan
  Irbesartan
  Candesartan
  Olmesartan
  Telmisartan
Renin inhibitor
  Aliskiren
Vasodilators
  Hydralazine
  Minoxidil

Diabetes

The two well-recognized forms of diabetes mellitus are called types 1 and 2. Type 1 diabetes is caused by a deficiency of insulin, the hormone secreted by the pancreas that allows the body to use sugar for energy. Patients with type 1 diabetes need to inject themselves with insulin, or high blood sugar, thirst, frequent urination, and weight loss will develop. Type 1 diabetes often develops in childhood or during early adult life. Type 2 diabetes most often develops in adulthood and is most common in overweight individuals. Unlike people with type 1 diabetes, these individuals produce insulin, but the insulin does not use blood sugar efficiently for energy. Type 2 diabetes is often managed by diet and pills that help lower blood sugar. Table 8-3 lists some of the pills used to control type 2 diabetes.

Diabetes has an important hereditary component. When both parents have diabetes, the development of diabetes in their children is almost certain. During the last 20 years there has been a dramatic increase in the frequency of diabetes—almost an epidemic. Some of this increase is explained by more frequent diagnosis. Much, however, may be related to the rising proportion of the population that is significantly overweight or frankly obese. Diabetes is especially common in these individuals. It is also more frequent among African Americans and Asians then Caucasians. Hypertension is more common in diabetics than in individuals who have normal blood sugar.

Individuals at risk for diabetes must carefully watch their weight and should follow a well-rounded diet that is relatively low in calories, carbohydrates, and salt.

Heart Disease

The heart is responsible for pumping blood into the arteries that supply the brain with blood. A variety of different cardiac conditions

TABLE 8-3 Agents Used to Treat Type 2 Diabetes Organized by Class

Biguanides
  Metformin
Sulfonylureas
  Tolbutamide
  Chlorpropamide
  Glyburide
  Glipizide
  Gliclazide
Meglitinides
  Repaglinide
  Nateglinide
Thiazolidinediones
  Pioglitazone
  Rosiglitazone
  Troglitazone
Glucagon-like peptide-1 agonists (subcutaneous)
  Exenatide
  Liraglutide
Alpha-glucosidase inhibitors
  Acarbose
  Miglitol
Dipeptidyl peptidase-4 inhibitors
  Sitagliptin
  Saxagliptin
  Vildagliptin
Insulin

place individuals at risk for developing strokes. Chapter 3 includes a description of the heart and its anatomy (see Figure 3.1).

Congenital Heart Disease

As described in Chapter 6, in some individuals the heart has formed abnormally during fetal development. Separation of the two sides of the heart may be incomplete and the heart valves or heart muscle may be malformed. Defects in the septum that divides the right heart chambers that pump blood into the lungs from the left heart chambers that supply blood to the rest of the body (atrial and ventricular septal defects, and patent foramen ovale) are relatively common, and can predispose to stroke. During birth, since babies' lungs do not function and do not breathe air, a hole exists through the upper chambers, the atria, that allows blood to go through the mother's circulatory system for oxygenation. At birth this oval-shaped hole (called the foramen ovale because of its shape) usually closes, but in about 30 percent of individuals it does not fully close. Figure 5-5 shows the heart structures and the septum between the left and right atria and ventricles—the location for various congenital defects that predispose people to stroke.

Heart Valve Disease

The valves in the heart ensure that blood is pumped in the correct direction and does not flow backwards from the ventricles into the atria, or from the pulmonary arteries and aorta into the ventricles. After the various chambers have contracted and expelled their contents, the valves close behind the contractions. Chapter 3 includes a discussion of the heart valves and their locations. Heart valves can become thickened, causing narrowing of the outflow tract (valvular stenosis), or can become leaky, allowing blood to pass in the reverse direction (valvular insufficiency). A variety of different valve diseases predispose to stroke: congenitally malformed valves, rheumatic fever and rheumatic heart disease, valve infections and inflammations, and degenerative thickening and scarring of the valves. Some patients eventually have their diseased heart valves replaced by prosthetic valves made from animal tissues or synthetic materials. Clots and infections can form on abnormal heart valves. These materials can break off and embolize to the brain, causing brain ischemia and infarction. Malfunctioning valves often lead to heart failure if not repaired or treated medically.

Heart Damage Related to Coronary Artery Disease

Loss of blood flow to a portion of the heart causes loss of heart muscle: a kind of stroke that affects the heart, a *myocardial infarction*, often referred to as a heart attack. The resulting loss of effective pumping function can cause heart failure and allow clots to form in the heart that can be ejected and reach the brain.

Abnormal Heart Rhythms

When the heart contracts irregularly and rapidly, it cannot efficiently expel the blood that is delivered to it. The most common **arrhythmia** is atrial fibrillation. This is a very common condition that increases in frequency with age. Inefficient contraction can lead to clots forming in the atria, which can be ejected and travel to the brain. Drugs can be prescribed in an attempt to restore and maintain normal heart rhythm. Sometimes electrical stimulation (defibrillation) is used to return the rhythm to normal. Studies have shown that prescribing anticoagulant drugs (warfarin, dabigatran, apixaban, and rivaroxaban) can greatly reduce the risk of stroke in individuals with atrial fibrillation.

High Cholesterol and Abnormalities of Blood Lipids

Lipids are derived from fats that are eaten or stored in the body. The body also can make lipids from other nutrients. High blood cholesterol levels are well known as an important risk factor for coronary artery disease. High cholesterol levels promote formation of plaques in arteries supplying the heart, limbs, and brain. Cholesterol and other lipids circulate in the blood attached to lipoproteins. There are two main forms of lipoproteins in the blood: HDL, which is known as the so-called good cholesterol, and LDL, which is known as the so-called bad cholesterol. Low levels of HDL and high levels of LDL are risk factors for heart disease and stroke. An increase in triglycerides can also promote plaque formation and predispose people to strokes. High blood levels of another lipid substance, lipoprotein-a, has also been associated with an increased frequency of stroke and coronary artery disease.

Individuals who have family members with high cholesterol levels are more likely than others also to have high blood lipids. Recognizing lipid abnormalities early in life can lead to their effective lowering by diet, exercise, and sometimes pills. It is important for individuals to know their levels of cholesterol and other blood lipids. Doctors can order lipid analyses that measure the amounts of the various types of lipid substances in your blood. High blood cholesterol and other lipid abnormalities can be lowered with the various medicines shown in Table 8-4. Some pills have more effects

TABLE 8-4 Drugs Used to Reduce High Blood Lipid Levels and to Reduce Atherosclerotic Plaque Formation

Statins
    Atorvastatin (Lipitor)
    Simvasatin (Zocor)
    Pravastatin (Pravachol)
    Fluvastatin (Lescol)
    Lovastatin (Mevacor)
    Rosuvastatin (Crestor)
Resins
    Cholestyramine (Questran)
    Colestipol (Colestid)
    Colesevelam (Welchol)
Niacin
Fibrates
    Gemfibrozil (Lopid)
    Fenofibrate (Tricor)
    Clofibrate (Atromid-S)
Omega-3 fatty acids (fish oil)

on certain lipid elements than other drugs and sometimes doctors prescribe combinations of these drugs.

Some of the medicines used to lower cholesterol, especially the class of drugs called statins, have additional functions that can limit the risk of strokes. Statins act on the lining cells of blood vessels (the endothelium) to limit the formation of atherosclerotic plaques. Even when blood cholesterol is normal, statins can prevent the buildup of plaques and may even reduce their size. Some physicians prescribe statin drugs for patients with strokes and for individuals with plaques who have not yet had strokes—even when their cholesterol levels are normal—to reduce plaque development and to enhance plaque reabsorption. Statins may also have a protective effect on the brain, increasing its resistance to reductions in blood flow. Studies show that high doses of statins (e.g., 80 mg of atorvastatin daily) are more effective in stroke prevention than low doses.

Most statins are best taken at night since they decrease absorption of lipids eaten during the day. Statins can cause some muscle cramping and discomfort, but serious muscle injury is quite rare (occurring in less than 1 percent of users).

Obesity

Being significantly overweight is a major risk factor for a number of medical conditions that pose a risk for stroke. Heavier people are more likely to have high blood pressure, diabetes, and high blood cholesterol. These conditions often occur together. The components of this so-called metabolic syndrome are obesity, high blood sugar, elevated blood cholesterol, and high blood pressure. Obesity is related to genetic factors and lifestyle. Overeating and inactivity clearly predispose to weight gain, but obesity is more related to how much you eat rather than what you eat. A well-rounded diet, relatively low in calories and salt, and regular exercise are the best antidotes to becoming or remaining overweight. Individuals with elevated blood pressures, large waistlines, blood lipid abnormalities, or who have a family history of close relatives with heart disease or stroke should be instructed about aggressive lifestyle changes and prescription medications to reduce their risk of developing diabetes, stroke, and heart disease.

Other Medical Illnesses and Conditions

Many medical conditions can be complicated by strokes. Cancer, AIDS, serious infections, and inflammatory diseases such as ulcerative colitis and Crohn's disease in the intestines, rheumatoid arthritis, systemic lupus erythematosus (often just called lupus), and others change the body's clotting functions and so increase the chance of clots developing within the arteries that supply the brain. Individuals who have a variety of kidney diseases have a higher than average frequency of stroke. Some kidney disease is caused by vascular conditions that also affect the brain. In estimating an individual's risk of stroke, it is useful to examine the urine for protein, estimate the glomerular filtration rate, and measure blood urine nitrogen and creatinine levels.

Blood Conditions

Abnormalities of the cells that circulate within the blood (red blood cells, white blood cells, and platelets) and of the liquid portion of the blood can cause excessive clotting or bleeding. Too many red blood cells (polycythemia) and a high percentage of the blood composed of red blood cells (high hematocrit) increase the thickness (viscosity) of the blood, causes slowed and sluggish blood flow, and predisposes to excess clotting, especially when individuals become dehydrated. Many older individuals have low fluid intakes. Severe anemia (very low red blood cell count and low hematocrit) is also a risk factor for stroke, and leukemia can also be associated with excess clotting or bleeding. Blood platelet abnormalities are also a very important cause of disease. A very high platelet count (thrombocytosis) leads to clotting and slow blood flow through vessels; a very low platelet count (thrombocytopenia) can cause spontaneous bleeding, sometimes within or around the brain.

A number of protein substances within the blood play a very important role in clotting. These substances protect against excess bleeding should a blood vessel be injured or cut. Some substances inhibit clotting (antithrombin III, protein C, and protein S), while other blood components (usually referred to as blood factors II, VII, VIII, IX, and X) stimulate clotting when activated. A deficiency in antithrombin III, or proteins C or S, either due to a congenital or acquired deficiency, can cause excessive clotting. Deficiencies of blood **coagulation** factors often cause excess bleeding. The best known such deficiency is hemophilia, which is caused by a deficiency of antihemophilic globulin (blood factor VIII). Two hereditary abnormalities—the presence of Leiden factor 5 (a deficiency of activated Protein C) and a prothrombin (factor II) gene mutation—are recognized as important but infrequent causes of increased blood clotting.

Pregnancy, Oral Contraceptives, and Sex Hormones

During and after pregnancy (postpartum), women have increased blood clotting potential. This increased tendency prevents bleeding from the uterus and helps maintain the placenta and the pregnancy, but raises the risk that leg veins and other vessels could develop clots. The pregnant uterus compresses veins that drain through the abdomen, which increases the tendency for leg vein clotting. The frequency of stroke is also increased, sometimes related to clotting of veins within the head. Users of oral contraceptive drugs composed of female hormones also have a slightly increased stroke frequency. The higher the dose, the greater the risk; low-estrogen drugs pose only a small risk. The presence of other potential risk factors such as smoking, migraine, and hypertension compound the stroke risk of using oral contraceptives. While it was once thought that female hormone replacement after menopause with estrogens, or estrogens and progesterones, helped prevent heart disease and stroke, recent studies suggest that these hormones are not protective and instead may increase the risk of stroke and coronary artery disease, depending somewhat on when they are prescribed. The use of male hormones to increase muscle mass and strength is also associated with an increased risk of vascular disease. Such use should be reserved only for those men whose bodies are deficient in these hormones. Some women take high doses of male hormones to change their appearance to look more masculine and less feminine, which also increases their risk of stroke.

Behavior and Lifestyle

Smoking

Cigarette smoking is strongly related to a higher risk of stroke and to increased narrowing and plaque formation in the arteries of the neck and head. The increased stroke risk applies to middle-aged and older individuals, to men and women, and especially to young people. The amount and duration of smoking are both important. In one study of young adults (aged 15–45 years) in Iowa, a smoker was 1.6 times more likely to have a stroke than a nonsmoker. Smoking was one of the most important risk factors among college students who later developed ischemic strokes. The length of time that someone has smoked and the number of packs that they smoked per day influences the development of atherosclerosis in the arteries that supply the brain and the heart. Smokers who stop smoking have less risk of stroke and heart attacks than those who continue to smoke. Smoking adds risk when other factors such as hypertension, diabetes, and the use of oral contraceptives are present.

Physical Inactivity

"Use it or lose it" is an adage that most people believe has some validity. Put a car, especially an old one, in a garage and fail to drive it for a while, and it may never be the same. Similarly, many body functions are so well coordinated that lack of use causes abilities and structures to wither with disuse. Regular exercise helps preserve a healthful weight, improve or maintain good heart function, reduce high blood pressure, and improve some blood lipid abnormalities. Physical exercise need not be rigorous to be healthy. Walking, swimming, and gardening are excellent physical activities if performed regularly.

Drugs

Illicit drugs, especially cocaine and methamphetamine (speed), have become a very important and frequent cause of both brain ischemia and brain hemorrhage in young and middle-aged adults. Crack cocaine is especially dangerous and causes sudden increases in blood pressure and contraction of brain blood vessels. Amphetamines similarly raise blood pressure abruptly and cause brain hemorrhages. Heroin injected through the veins can cause brain and spinal cord strokes. Some people mash up pills meant for oral use and inject them intravenously. Particles of substances such as talc that are used for fillers in these pills can reach the brain and the eyes, leading to strokes and vision loss.

Prescription drugs, even when given appropriately, can also become risk factors for strokes. Anticoagulant drugs (coumadin, heparin and dabigatran, apixaban, rivaroxaban) can cause bleeding into the brain and other organs, especially if the intensity of anticoagulation (as usually measured in the case of coumadin by the international normalized ratio) is higher than desired. Aspirin and other so-called antiplatelet drugs such as clopidogrel, ticlopidine, and to a lesser extent dipyridamole, can also cause bleeding. Last, some drugs used to treat cancer and leukemia can cause excess clotting or bleeding and so lead to stroke.

Migraine

Migraine is one of the most misunderstood medical conditions. When people on the street are asked about their understanding of migraine, they almost always define it as frequent, extremely severe, blinding headaches. In fact, migraine can occur even without headache. When headaches do occur they can also be slight and infrequent.

Migraine is a hereditary condition that most often begins in early life and is more frequent in girls and women than in boys and men. During a migraine attack, arteries can narrow considerably, causing dizziness, disturbed vision, abnormal sensations, and other neurologic symptoms. Arteries can also dilate, meaning that their diameter widens. This widening presses on nerve endings on the outside of the arteries, causing headache (often on just one side of the head) and throbbing. Vomiting is also common. One of the books in the series published by the American Academy of Neurology considers and explains migraine in detail.

During a migraine attack, vomiting and decreased fluid intake are common. Blood platelets are also activated. The dehydration and increased clotting tendency can lead to clots forming in already narrowed arteries, leading to the development of a so-called migrainous stroke in the portion of the brain supplied by the blocked artery. Because dehydration raises this risk, doctors often urge migraine patients to continue to drink adequately during a migraine. Doctors often prescribe aspirin and drugs to prevent or minimize vasoconstriction and to prevent migraine in some patients.

Physical Activities

An increasing number of arterial injuries come from physical injuries. Head injuries can cause bleeding within and around the brain.

Automobile and sports injuries can cause tearing of arteries within the neck and head that lead to strokes. These injuries are usually related to sudden head and neck movements that stretch the neck arteries. Neck manipulations are often performed by health care practitioners for neck pain and headache. Blood vessel tears (dissections) can develop after neck manipulation and can lead to serious sometimes fatal strokes.

Blood Test Markers

Doctors have started to place emphasis on the results of various blood tests that could indicate a heightened risk for stroke or vascular disease. These are listed in Table 8-5.

High and very low hematocrit levels, polycythemia, and abnormally high platelet counts increase the risk of brain ischemia. Very low platelet counts (thrombocytopenia) increase the risk of bleeding and brain hemorrhage. Fibrinogen is a component of blood clots and plaques within arteries. High fibrinogen levels increase the risk of brain ischemia. High values of **homocysteine** and C-reactive protein (CRP) increase the risk of atherosclerosis in arteries that supply the heart, limbs, and brain. Low levels of HDL and high levels of LDL increase the risk of atherosclerosis.

TABLE 8-5 Blood Tests Sometimes Used to Indicate Stroke Risk

Hematocrit
Platelet count
Homocysteine
C-reactive protein
Antiphospholipid antibodies
Fibrinogen
Cholesterol, HDL, and LDL
Triglycerides

Phospholipids are present in some blood components and in blood vessels. Some individuals develop antibodies to phospholipids. High levels of antiphospholipid antibodies lead to an increased frequency of miscarriages, strokes, leg vein clotting, and migraine.

Ultrasound and Other Imaging Tests

Doctors may order ultrasound and brain and vascular imaging tests in individuals who they believe are at risk of having a stroke. Often this is because they have risk factors such as hypertension, diabetes, high cholesterol, as previously discussed in this chapter. Sometimes the tests are ordered because doctors hear a noise (often referred to using the French word for noise, bruit, as described in Chapter 7) when listening to the neck arteries. Sometimes the tests are done in patients being examined for other medical problems, such as headache or suspected tumor.

I discuss these tests at length next in Chapter 9, which describes patient evaluation. Brain images may show unsuspected stroke-related damage or vascular malformations. Vascular imaging tests can show plaques in arteries in the neck or brain or in the aorta. Blocked or narrowed arteries, aneurysms, and vascular malformations may also be found.

Even though the patient with these abnormalities may not have symptoms, these tests can guide treatment to prevent stroke.

Comments on Diet

Health is not determined only by what you eat. Nevertheless many individuals are intensely focused on dietary intake as the way to prevent the development of disease. Research on the relationship between the intake of various foods and disease is particularly difficult. To show that a given food substance either prevents or contributes to the development of a given medical condition, researchers prefer to have everything else (intake of all other foods, genetics, behavior, disease, etc.) remain the same. The only variable should be the food substance being tested. Unfortunately, in real life there are many, many other variables that cannot readily be controlled for.

The American Heart Association and other medical organizations agree on some nutritional recommendations. Do not overeat. Limit salt intake. Fruits, vegetables, and whole grains are good foods to eat. Fish and fish oils help prevent vascular disease. Some information suggests that certain foods may help prevent stroke, heart attacks, and vascular diseases. These recommended substances include soy products, grape products, tea, walnuts and almonds, and tomato products.

Chapter 9

How Can Doctors Tell What Caused the Stroke? What Tests Are Used to Evaluate Individuals Who May Have Had a Stroke?

History of the Events and Symptoms

The patient's description of the symptoms and the events that occurred is of utmost importance. Chapter 7 includes a description of the most common general and neurologic symptoms. The description of the event(s) is especially important when the symptoms were transient, since only the patient's account can provide information about the nature of the abnormality. Doctors are taught that the history (what the patient and others tell them) is the most important key to an accurate diagnosis. Doctors can glean much about the nature and cause of the symptoms when a detailed history of the account and the past medical history are available. Very important clues that indicate *where* the stroke is in the brain and *what* caused it come from the history that the doctor takes from the patient and the results of the physical and neurologic examinations. Because of the publicity that new technologies have received, many patients think that history taking and physical examinations have been replaced by scans, but this is certainly not true. Examining patients is the only way to know what they can and cannot do.

In Table 9-1, I list some of the key questions asked during the history taking for the acute event. Although the questions are aimed at the patient, often others who have accompanied the patient can also provide useful information, especially if they were with the

TABLE 9-1 Sample Questions about the Acute Event

What were you doing before and at the onset of the symptoms?
Was the onset very sudden or did the symptoms gradually develop?
After the symptoms were first noticed, did they improve, stay the
  same, or worsen? Did they ever go away for a time?
Did you have a headache before, during, or after the onset of the
  symptoms?
Did you vomit or have a change in your state of alertness?
If the symptoms were temporary, how long did they last?
Did you ever have similar symptoms or attacks? If so, when? Were the
  symptoms the same as the current event or different?

patient during the event(s). When the patient cannot communicate well, the account of others is crucial.

In general, ischemic strokes due to embolism are most often maximal at onset, while ischemic strokes due to a local process in the vessels can fluctuate and develop more gradually and are often preceded by TIAs. Subarachnoid hemorrhages invariably cause headache at onset. Hemorrhages in the brain often cause symptoms that worsen over a few minutes.

Past medical history is also helpful in diagnosis. The presence of past strokes and other cardiovascular events, such as hypertension and heart attacks, provides clues to the most likely process that caused the current event. Since other medical conditions can predispose to strokes, they also should be discussed. Information about the history of vascular disease and risk factors in the patient's family can also be useful. Table 9-2 lists some of the past history that is often pursued. Quantification is important; hospital charts and doctors' records could list hypertension, but not include details or levels. Consider two different individuals: one patient who once had slightly high blood pressure, and another whose blood pressure has been very high and uncontrolled for years. The second patient's

---

TABLE 9-2 Past Medical and Social History of Importance

---

1. Hypertension? For how long? How severe? Treated with medications? How well controlled?
2. Diabetes? How treated: diet, oral agents, insulin? When was it first diagnosed? Complications? Eyes, nerves, kidneys?
3. High cholesterol? Can you give me the numbers? How treated? For how long?
4. Overweight? If so, how much and for how long?
5. Physical activities and exercise? What kind? How often?
6. Past medical conditions? Heart attacks, claudication of the legs while walking, arthritis, inflammatory bowel disease, past excess clotting or bleeding?
7. Smoking? For how long? Now smoking or stopped? If stopped, how long ago?
8. Alcohol intake? How much and for how long?

---

stroke risk is considerably higher than the first patient, but the two very different risk profiles are often both recorded simply as "hypertension."

The Physical Examination

General and neurologic physical examinations tell doctors where the problem is in the brain, the presence and severity of the neurologic deficit, and the presence of cardiovascular abnormalities. The examination includes measuring the blood pressure, taking the pulse, listening to the heart, and feeling and listening over the blood vessels in the arms and neck. Neurologic testing includes assessments of alertness, speech, memory, vision; the strength, feeling, coordination, and reflexes in all four limbs; and watching the patient walk. A score that reflects the severity of the dysfunction is often estimated. The most commonly used score is generated from the

National Institutes of Health Stroke Scale. I discussed in Chapter 7 the examination findings that doctors look for in patients suspected of having had a stroke.

Radiology and Other Laboratory Testing

The laboratory testing that doctors order to evaluate patients depends very much on the nature of the symptoms and signs in each patient and on their underlying stroke risk factors. Of course, each patient suspected of stroke may not undergo all of the tests available. I aim simply to familiarize readers with the evaluation and testing process. Doctors are now able to find out, safely and quickly, whether a person has had a stroke and whether a patient's stroke is due to hemorrhage or ischemia. They can also determine where and how much of the brain has been damaged, and the presence, nature, and severity of any abnormalities affecting the blood vessels that supply the brain. Tests also can show if heart or blood abnormalities were the primary or contributing cause of the stroke. Knowing exactly what is wrong with the stroke patient allows selection of the best treatment. Stroke patients and their families will want to become familiar with the tests available so that they can understand what has or has not been done to investigate the stroke and the blood vessels.

Brain Imaging

There are two general types of brain imaging tests: **computed tomography (CT)** and **magnetic resonance imaging (MRI)**. CT uses ordinary X-rays and computers to make thin slices through different levels of the brain. The technique is like slicing a loaf of bread. Each slice contains a picture of the brain structures present at that level. MRI uses magnetic energy to create images of the brain. Both tests are safe and painless. Each requires the patient to place their head into a machine; with MRI, much of the body may also be enclosed. Patients must remain still if the machines are to be able to make clear, high-quality images. The MRI machine makes noise, and many people who are claustrophobic have difficulty staying still in the machine. MRI produces more different image sections of the brain and generates images at different angles: from the top to the bottom (coronal), along the long axis of the brain (axial), and from side to side (sagittal). To generate a more detailed brain image, doctors may order an intravenous injection of a substance that adds contrast to the images obtained. With CT this is usually an iodine-containing substance; for MRI, a chemical containing gadolinium is used for contrast enhancement. Occasionally patients have an allergic response to these contrast substances, especially to the dye used for CT contrast.

CT and MRI allow doctors to distinguish brain hemorrhages from infarctions. They can also show whether bleeding has occurred in the areas within the skull but outside of the brain—in the subarachnoid, subdural, or epidural spaces. (These locations were discussed and depicted in Chapter 4.) On CT scans, hemorrhages appear white and infarcts appear gray or black, making it quite easy to distinguish the two main stroke categories. Figure 9-1 is an image from a CT scan of patient Robert H. that shows a brain infarct involving the right cerebral hemisphere. Figure 9-2 contains a CT scan of Claire H. that shows a small brain infarct within the left cerebral hemisphere. The infarct appears darker than the surrounding normal brain. Adjacent to the CT scan in Figure 9-2 is a diffusion-weighted image (DWI) from the MRI examination of Claire H. that shows the infarct (in white) more clearly than the CT scan. Figure 9-3 is the CT scan from Tom M. that shows a cerebellar brain hemorrhage. The region of bleeding appears whiter than the surrounding tissue. Figure 9-4 is an MRI image from a patient whose brain infarct involves the same general region as that shown in the CT scan of Figure 9-1. Figure

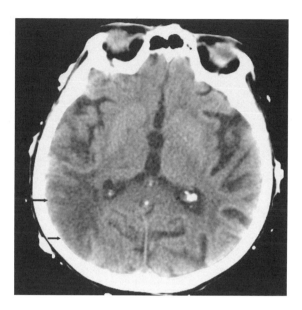

FIGURE 9-1 A CT scan showing a portion of the large brain infarct in Robert H. The black arrows point to the black area that represents the infarct within the right temporal lobe.

9-5a–c includes MRI images from other patients with brain infarcts. Figures 9-6a and b shows a brain hemorrhage imaged by CT and MRI. CT shows hemorrhages as localized white areas, while T2*-weighted MRI images show brain hemorrhages as localized black regions.

There are a number of different types of images that can be obtained using MRI. DWI images effectively show areas of infarction even minutes after they develop. Blood perfusion can be studied using perfusion-weighted images that are obtained by infusing a contrast agent and following its passage through the brain. Brain perfusion can also be studied using CT scanners. Other MRI images, especially T2*-weighted scans best show areas of bleeding.

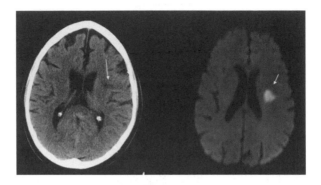

FIGURE 9-2 A CT scan (left) and an MRI scan (right) in patient Claire H. The white arrow in the CT scan points to a dark area that represents the infarct within the left cerebral hemisphere. The same infarct is shown on the MRI scan as a well-defined white lesion.

Brain images not only show whether the lesion is a hemorrhage or infarct; they also show where the abnormality is located, how large and extensive it is, and whether there is brain swelling and pressure inside of the head caused by the infarct or hemorrhage. In some patients with temporary symptoms of brain ischemia, CT and MRI can appear normal, indicating that the brain has not been irreversibly damaged—that is, not yet infarcted. Knowing where the abnormality is in the brain allows doctors to know which blood vessels supply the abnormal region. These vessels can then be checked for abnormalities.

Making Images of the Blood Vessels and Determining Blood Flow

Having identified the stroke-related abnormalities in the brain, doctors then test the arteries that supply the injured brain. Pictures of the arteries (angiograms) can be created using a CT scanner. These **CT angiograms** (CTAs) are made by injecting an iodine-containing dye

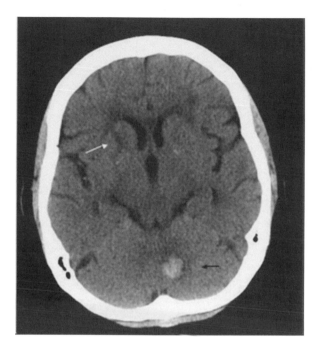

FIGURE 9-3 CT scan in patient Tom M. The small black arrow near the bottom of the scan points to a recent hemorrhage in the left cerebellum. The hemorrhage appears as a well-defined round lighter area. The white arrow at the upper left side of the scan points to an old infarct adjacent to the right caudate nucleus. The infarct appears as a dark arc-shaped zone.

and then taking pictures rapidly as the dye goes through the arteries and veins throughout the brain. **Magnetic resonance angiograms** (MRA) can be made without injecting dye. Blood moving through arteries and veins will appear in the image if the settings on the MRI machine are changed to capture these vascular structures instead of the brain. MRA can be performed at the same time as MRI and CTA examinations can be done at the same time as CT. Figure 9-7 contains two MRA scans. Figure 9-7a is an MRA examination of Tom M. that shows a right internal carotid artery occlusion and an

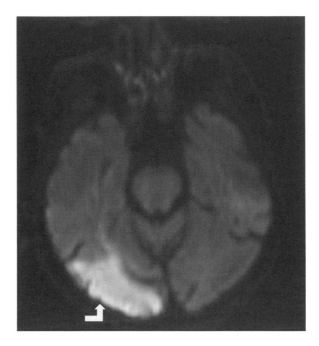

FIGURE 9-4 A DWI from an MRI showing a right temporal lobe infarct (large white arrow). Compare this MRI, which shows the infarct in white, with the CT scan in Fig 9-1 that shows a similarly located infarct as a gray-black area.

irregular plaque within the left internal carotid artery. The MRA in Figure 9-7b shows a minor region of narrowing in the basilar artery. Figure 9-8 contains two CTA examinations. Figure 9-8a is a CTA that should be compared with the MRA in Figure 9-7b. The basilar artery shows a region within the beginning of the artery that has no flow, indicating very severe narrowing or occlusion. Figures 9-8b and 9-8c are images from a CTA examination of Elaine S. They show a sharp cutoff of the middle cerebral artery. The image in 9-8c has been modified to show the arteries more clearly.

Ultrasound, sometimes called **Doppler ultrasound** after Christian Doppler (who described how the frequency of sound

(a)

(b)

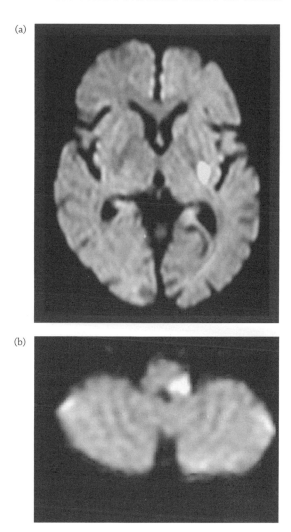

FIGURE 9-5 a. A T2-weighted MRI, that shows a small, localized, ovoid infarct in the left internal capsule on the right side of the figure. b. A DWI from an MRI that shows an infarct in the lateral medulla as a discrete bright white region. c. A T2-weighted MRI that shows a very large infarct in the right cerebellum that extends into the brainstem. (Continued)

(c)

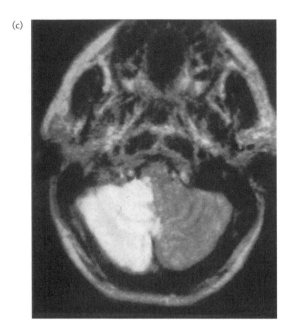

FIGURE 9-5 (Continued)

and light waves can change relative to the motion of their source as a result of his astronomy studies), is another very effective way to safely study arterial blood flow. The testing is done by placing a small probe over blood vessels in the neck, and over the eyes, back of the head, and sides of the head. The ultrasound information is relayed into an analyzing machine that creates pictures of the vessels and also calculates the speed of blood moving through the blood vessels directly under the probes. The ultrasound findings can show if an artery is normal, narrowed, or completely blocked. Figure 9-9a illustrates a neck ultrasound examination.

So-called duplex ultrasound scans of the neck create images and sound curves of the carotid and vertebral arteries in the neck. Some

(a)

(b)

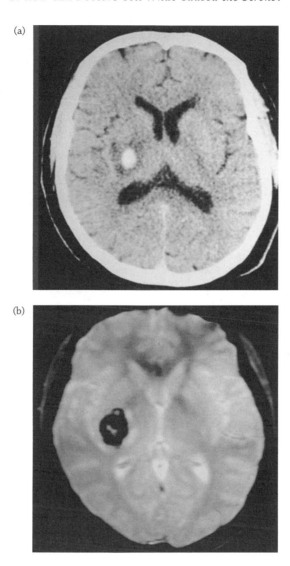

FIGURE 9-6 a. A CT scan that shows a small, recent hemorrhage in the right basal ganglia as a small white round region with a surrounding gray zone that represents edema. b. A T2*-weighted MRI that shows a similarly located hemorrhage as a well-defined black area.

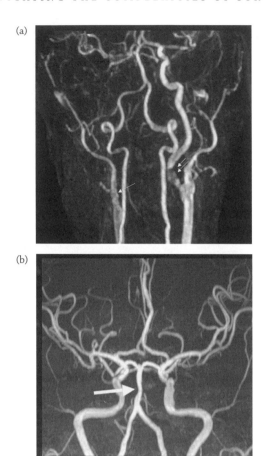

FIGURE 9-7   a. An MRA of the neck and head arteries in patient Robert H. The single white arrow on the left of the figure points to the region where the right internal carotid artery should begin. The right internal carotid artery is occluded, so it cannot be seen above this region in the neck. The left internal carotid artery contains an irregular plaque (two white arrows) that is shown as a darker irregular region within the first part of the artery. b. An MRA scan of the arteries in the head. There is a localized region of slight narrowing (white arrow) within the basilar artery that represents a plaque. In this MRA both Internal carotid arteries are shown and are symmetrical, in contrast to the missing right internal carotid artery in Figure 9-7a.

(a)

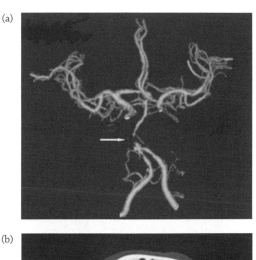

(b)

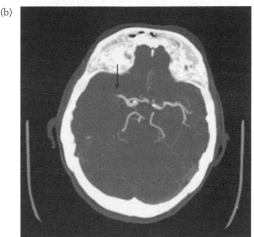

FIGURE 9-8   a. A subtracted image from a CTA examination that shows a nearly complete occlusion of the basilar artery (arrow). Blood flow is easily seen below and above the zone of no flow. b. An image of the brain filmed during a CTA examination of Elaine S. The right middle cerebral artery abruptly ends (black arrow). Contrast this amputated artery with its normal counterpart, the left middle cerebral artery, shown on the opposite side of the brain. c. An image from the same CTA examination shown in 9-8b. The brain has been subtracted. The occlusion is seen very clearly (long white arrow). (Continued)

(c)

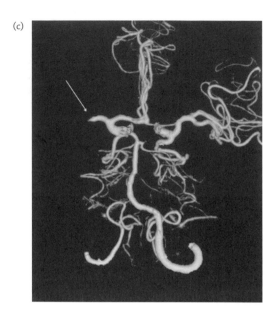

FIGURE 9-8 (Continued)

laboratories use **transcranial Doppler ultrasound** (TCD) to examine blood flow in the arteries inside of the head (see Figure 9-9b). In this technique, small probes are placed over the eyes, the back of the neck, and the temples—places where the skull is absent or thin. Blood flow velocities in the various arteries within the skull are also checked for narrowing, occlusion, or abnormally increased or decreased blood flow. When an artery in the neck is narrowed or blocked, TCD of the main branches of that artery in the head can reflect the impact of the disease in the neck vessels on blood flow to the threatened region of the brain.

All of the brain and vascular imaging tests described are quite safe and can be performed quickly either inside or outside of hospitals. The strategy used to locate the blood vessel abnormality is similar to that used by a plumber trying to discover why water does not flow to the second-floor sink on one side of the house. The

(a)

(b)

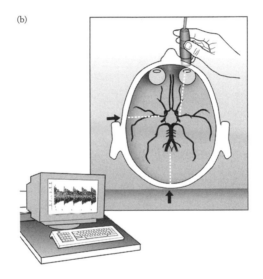

FIGURE 9-9 a. A drawing of an ultrasound examination of the neck. The probe is held over one of the carotid arteries and is attached to a computer monitor, which depicts the arterial structures beneath the probe. b. A drawing showing a perspective looking down from above the patient's head. The eyes and nose are facing towards the top of the picture. A probe is placed on the right eye. The monitor shows the pulse spectrum in the arteries behind the eye. The brain is removed and a drawing of the location of the arteries is shown within the uncapped skull.

problem with that sink must be within the water system that supplies it, including the water tank and its outflow and the pipes leading to that sink.

When these so-called noninvasive tests do not give enough information about the diseased arteries, physicians may order a catheter angiogram to be performed by a radiology or neurologic interventional specialist. This test is more invasive and carries a small but definite risk of complications. When doctors order this test, they judge that the information needed is important enough to warrant the small risk. Some treatments on blocked vessels, aneurysms, and vascular malformations are delivered through the feeding arteries. In these cases, vascular access to the artery is required for treatment and angiograms are needed to monitor the effect of treatment. The interventional specialist places a catheter in one of the arteries of the thighs or arms and threads it under visual control, using a monitoring fluoroscopic screen, into the arteries in the neck. Dye is then injected, and a series of rapid-fire X-rays are taken that show the dye as it passes through the arteries and veins. This creates a cast-like picture of the inside of the arteries that can show areas of narrowing or blockage, aneurysms, and vascular malformations. At times the specialist performing the angiography can give treatment to open narrowed or blocked arteries or to obliterate vascular malformations or aneurysms.

Complications of catheter angiography most often consist of an allergic response to the dye, inadvertent injury to an artery into which the catheter is placed, or dislodging a plaque or clot from an artery that then passes into the brain. In the hands of most well-trained and experienced specialists, these complications occur in only one or two patients in 100 and the great majority of complications are minor and temporary. Still, doctors try to avoid catheter angiography if the preliminary tests provide enough information. The more the doctor knows about the patient's abnormalities, the better they can choose treatment.

All of the patients discussed in Chapter 1 had brain imaging that clarified the location and nature of their strokes. Claire H.'s MRA showed a dissection of her left internal carotid artery in the neck. CT and MRI scans had shown a small brain infarct in the region of the left middle cerebral artery. Robert H.'s CT (Figure 9-1) and MRI (Figure 9-4) scans showed an infarct in his right cerebral hemisphere. His MRA examination (Figure 9-7a) showed an occluded internal carotid artery in his neck. The left internal carotid artery contained an irregular atherosclerotic plaque. Note that the right internal carotid artery is not visualized. Compare the images to Figure 9-7b, an MRA that shows both internal carotid arteries. A duplex ultrasound confirmed that the carotid artery was occluded in the neck. TCD showed low blood flow velocities over the right eye. Elaine S.'s CTA (Figures 9-8b and c) showed that her right middle cerebral artery was blocked by the embolus that had originated in her heart as a result of atrial fibrillation. Tom M.'s CT scan showed a small cerebellar hemorrhage; it also showed evidence of prior brain infarcts related to his untreated hypertension. In his case, I did not feel it required vascular imaging, since the cause was clearly uncontrolled hypertension.

Heart Tests

Heart testing is useful in almost all patients with stroke. The heart often acts as a source of clot formation, and clots and fragments of heart valves can break off and embolize to the brain, causing strokes. Individuals who have narrowing of the large arteries in the neck that supply blood to the brain often also have narrowing of the arteries that supply the heart muscle (the coronary arteries).

Electrocardiograms (EKGs) have long been used to study the heart. They show the rate at which the heart is beating (the pulse rate) and identify heart rhythm abnormalities. This simple, familiar test can also show the evidence of past heart attacks. Robert H's electrocardiogram showed evidence of a previous heart attack, but his heart rhythm was normal. Elaine S.'s EKG showed atrial fibrillation. In Tom M., the EKG showed evidence of enlargement of the left-side heart muscle (left ventricular hypertrophy) caused by his hypertension. Claire H. had a normal EKG.

Ultrasound of the heart (called **echocardiography**) can yield pictures of the various parts of the heart and their functioning. It is performed by a technician or a cardiologist, who places an ultrasound probe on the chest or has the patient swallow a string-like device containing an ultrasound probe that travels into the esophagus. Much of the heart can be seen better from the back through the esophagus than from the front. The cardiologist can see the heart valves, the upper heart chambers (atria), and the left and right ventricles. Sometimes saline bubbles are injected into an arm vein to see their passage through the heart. In patients who have atrial and ventricular septal defects and PFOs, the bubbles can pass from the right side of the heart to the left chambers. In Robert H. the echocardiogram showed a region of impaired contraction where he had had a myocardial infarction. In Elaine S., the echocardiogram showed a thrombus within the left atrium of the heart (Figure 9-10).

Studying the Electrical Activity of the Brain

By placing small electrodes over the scalp, doctors can record and study the electrical activity of the brain. This test is called an **electroencephalogram** (EEG). It is often used to distinguish between a TIA and a seizure arising from increased brain activity. Patients with seizures also can have temporary interruptions in their functions that can be difficult to distinguish from TIAs without an EEG. Strokes can occasionally cause injuries that

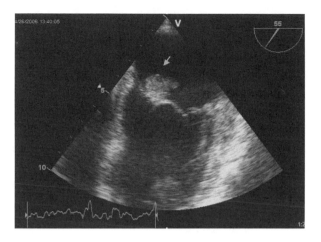

FIGURE 9-10

An image from an echocardiogram that shows a large thrombus (white arrow) within the left atrium of the heart.

induce abnormal electrical discharge, which leads patients to develop seizures.

Blood Tests

Blood tests are very important and are routinely performed in patients who either have had a stroke or who are suspected of having had a TIA or a stroke. I list the blood tests in Table 9-3. Of course not all of these tests will be ordered for every patient. Blood counts are routinely performed because amounts of all of the blood components (red and white blood cells and platelets) that are too high or too low can cause strokes and other medical problems. Some screening tests of blood coagulation are ordered, usually a prothrombin time and a platelet count. Only when these screening tests are abnormal, or when there is a strong indication of excess clotting or

TABLE 9-3 Blood Tests

Blood cell counts
  Red blood cells
  Hemoglobin and hematocrit
  White blood cells
  Differential count of the various types of white blood cells
    (polymorphonuclear cells, lymphocytes, monocytes, eosinophils,
    basophils)
  Platelets
Blood clotting tests
  Prothrombin time (PT)—often reported in terms of an interna-
    tional normalized ratio (INR)
  Accelerated partial thromboplastin time (APTT)
  Antithrombin III, protein C, protein S
  Leiden factor 5
  Prothrombin gene mutation
  Levels of blood factors II, VII, VIII, IX, X
  Lupus anticoagulant, anticardiolipin antibodies
Blood sugar
  Glycosylated hemoglobin- Hemoglobin A1C levels
Blood lipids
  Total cholesterol
  HDL and LDL
  Triglycerides
  Lipoprotein-a
Heart enzymes
  Creatine kinase
  cardiac (CK-MB) and brain (CK-BB) isoenzyme levels
  troponin levels
Kidney function
  Blood urea nitrogen (BUN)
  Creatinine
Liver function
  Bilirubin
  Alkaline phosphatase

TABLE 8-2 (continued)

Blood electrolytes
  Sodium
  Potassium
  Calcium
  Chloride
  Carbon dioxide (CO_2)
Homocysteine
Vitamin levels
  B_{12}
  Folic Acid
Inflammatory markers and antibodies
  Erythrocyte sedimentation rate (ESR)
  C-reactive protein (CRP)
  Fibrinogen
  Antiphospholipid antibodies
  Rheumatoid factor
  LE cells

excess bleeding in the clinical history, are further explorations of clotting abnormalities made. Most of the other tests are selectively ordered depending on the individual patient's risk factors and the nature of their stroke and their coexisting medical conditions.

Blood lipid tests are familiar to most people. They test the levels of cholesterol, triglycerides, and other lipoproteins in the blood because high levels of fats can promote atherosclerosis and plaque formation in arteries supplying the heart, brain, and limbs. Disorders of the kidneys, blood electrolytes, and the liver can cause or complicate strokes and are often measured in stroke patients. Cancers and a variety of inflammatory conditions can cause strokes; markers of inflammation and of other specific conditions are therefore occasionally measured in the blood.

Recently, doctors have showed that elevated levels of homocysteine, CRP, and fibrinogen, and very low levels of B_{12}, predispose patients to stroke, and these are often measured in patients thought to be at risk for stroke and/or heart disease and in those who have already had a stroke.

Centers specializing in stroke have the technology and test equipment, and individuals who are experienced in performing and interpreting the tests, on duty all of the time. Tests can and should be done quickly. Experienced neurologists can select the tests that are needed and appropriate for each patient. Some of the testing needs to be done more urgently in patients with stroke; other tests can be ordered later. The brain is probably our most important resource, and it must be protected from stroke-related damage. The brain is vulnerable; deprivation of needed energy can kill brain cells within minutes or a very few hours. As the saying goes, "Time = brain." The longer a region is deprived of normal blood flow and nutrients, the more likely it is that region will die. The faster ischemia is corrected, the better the chance of saving vital tissues. Whenever possible, patients must come to centers equipped to diagnose and treat them quickly, and doctors must investigate and treat the problem urgently.

Chapter 10

What Treatments Are Available to Treat Acute Stroke Patients?

Treatment depends very much on what is wrong with the individual patient. Better diagnostic technology such as MRI, CT, and ultrasound have made it much easier to precisely locate abnormalities and have greatly enhanced treatment. Newer medical, surgical, and radiological techniques have been developed over the past three decades that profoundly increase doctors' ability to treat patients with brain hemorrhages and brain ischemia. In this chapter, I discuss treatment in terms of the various problems patients present to doctors.

Acute Brain Ischemia

In treating patients with an acute ischemic stroke, there are three general treatment strategies: (1) quickly try to bring more blood to the regions that are lacking blood flow, (2) give medicines to reduce the chances of formation and spread of blood clots, and (3) modify risk factors to prevent recurrent strokes and/or heart attacks.

Opening Blocked Arteries

The most important strategy is to bring more blood to the threatened brain region. One way to do this is to reopen the blocked artery that supplies that territory. This tactic is called **reperfusion** because it involves restoring blood flow to regions of the brain that have recently been deprived of their normal blood supply. To explain, let's consider a situation that will be familiar to almost all readers: watering a wilting lawn. Bringing blood to a part of the brain that is undersupplied with it is similar to bringing water to dry areas of the lawn. Let's assume a hose that supplies a portion of the lawn with needed water becomes blocked. A number of strategies could be used to bring water to the dry area. You could try to unblock the hose by cutting it open and removing the obstruction (surgical endarterectomy); or by using a mechanical instrument like a rotary cutter to attempt to unblock the hose (angioplasty); or employing a different instrument to mechanically suck out the material blocking the hose (a clot-retrieval device); or by introducing a chemical compound, some type of drain cleaner, to dissolve the materials blocking the hose (thrombolysis). You also might want to make sure the hose does not get blocked again by placing a mechanical layer within the hose to strengthen it (stenting). Alternately, if you could not remove or dissolve the obstruction, you could create a detour around the blockage by attaching another piece of hose before and beyond the region of blockage to route flow around it (surgical bypass). You could also try to increase water flow in adjacent hoses to try and reach the dry places.

The advanced imaging technology discussed in Chapter 9 can help with decisions about reperfusion. Both CT and MRI can show brain regions that are already infarcted, and vascular imaging (CTA, MRA, ultrasound) can show if and where a feeding artery is blocked. This information can guide doctors in deciding whether the benefits outweigh the risks of reperfusion and the method of reperfusion that is most likely to be effective.

Thrombolysis

Doctors can use the identical strategies in patients with acute ischemic strokes who have blockage in arteries. **Thrombolysis** is the term used to describe chemical dissolution of clots that are blocking arteries. The most common thrombolytic drug now used is **tissue plasminogen activator (tPA)** but researchers are now exploring other potential agents. tPA and other thrombolytic drugs can be given either intravenously or by having a specialist place a catheter within the blocked artery to deliver the drug directly to the clot (referred to as intra-arterial delivery). To be effective, tPA must be given rather soon after stroke develops. Thrombolytic drugs can cause bleeding into the brain and into other organs. Thrombolysis is hazardous when the blood pressure is very high, when the patient's blood clotting system indicates a tendency for bleeding, and when the patient has had recent surgery or another intervention. It is not appropriate in every patient that is seen soon after stroke. When extensive brain infarction is already present and when arteries are not blocked, the risk of treatment may outweigh the potential benefit. Whether or not to use tPA and other thrombolytic drugs is a judgment call that depends on a number of different considerations for each individual patient. If no large artery is blocked, there is no reason to infuse thrombolytics. If a large area of brain is already infarcted, opening the supplying artery gains little and carries a risk of inducing bleeding and brain edema. The ideal situation for thrombolysis is an artery that has recently become blocked by an embolus with no or little brain infarction. In that circumstance intravenous tPA has a strong likelihood of being effective. Elaine S., the older woman who developed sudden-onset embolism from atrial fibrillation, was given tPA. After being examined and having CT and CTA examinations, she received the thrombolytic agent to try and open her occluded right middle cerebral artery.

Surgery

When surgeons can expose the blocked artery segment, they can operate directly on the artery to unblock it. This procedure is called an endarterectomy, because surgeons remove the inner portion of the artery (the endarterial region). Surgeons place a temporary clamp above and below the diseased segment. They then open it and remove the inner core of plaque and clot material. After the artery has been cleaned out, it is sewed back up and the clamps are removed. The process takes a half hour or less in most cases. Endarterectomies are usually feasible when the artery is severely narrowed but not totally blocked by clot. When a clot forms, it often blocks the artery and extends far beyond its origin, making it impossible to reopen the artery surgically. Endarterectomy is used almost entirely for blockage within the neck in the carotid and vertebral arteries. Most arteries that commonly become blocked within the head are not readily exposed for surgery.

If blocked arteries cannot be repaired directly, surgeons can reconstruct the blood flow channels by using various techniques. They can connect the part of an artery leading toward the head into another artery. Alternately they can bring another artery into a position next to the blocked artery and sew the two vessels together. They can take a segment of another vessel from a distant site and use it to detour around the blocked artery. Sometimes doctors will place a muscle or tissue from the abdomen onto the outside of the brain in an ischemic area and sew the tissue to the surface, encouraging ingrowth of blood vessels from the tissue into the brain. This is used mostly in an unusual disorder that affects young people called moyamoya disease (see Chapter 6).

Angioplasty and Stenting

Specialists can also use an instrument inserted within an artery to dilate and open the artery. This process, called **angioplasty,** can be used to open arteries within the neck and head, especially when those arteries are not readily accessible for surgery. Sometimes doctors use a stent after angioplasty to keep the artery open, or put in a stent without doing an angioplasty first. **Stents** are wire-mesh sleeves that, when expanded, can mechanically dilate the lumen of an artery and attempt to keep it open.

Mechanical Devices to Remove Clots

A number of devices are now available that can approach and remove blood clots within large arteries within the head. The devices are threaded through catheters to the near end of the occluding clot. Some of the devices spear the clot like a fishhook and hold it until it is withdrawn through the catheter. Other devices apply a vacuum effect to suck the clot out. Some devices work like removable stents to grab the clot while opening the artery. The **interventionalist** who performs the study will have a variety of different techniques that can be used, including applying a range of mechanical devices and using intra-arterial thrombolytic agents.

Maximizing Blood Flow

Beyond these techniques, it is also important to try to generally improve blood flow to the head. When an artery is blocked, flow to the ischemic zone and its surrounding tissues comes from other nearby arteries (called collateral circulation) that ordinarily do not directly supply that region. Ischemic brain tissue gives off chemicals that encourage ingrowth of collateral blood vessels to help take up the blood-flow slack. Doctors may try to boost this process by maintaining or slightly raising blood pressure, increasing the amount of body fluids, and decreasing the viscosity of the blood. In patients with very high blood pressure, lowering the blood pressure can increase blood flow. Treating very high blood sugar may also help with energy delivery.

Changing the Tendency of Blood to Clot

Another common strategy often used in patients with vessel narrowing, occlusion, or embolism is to use various drugs that reduce the body's tendency to form clots. The two categories of clot-preventing drugs are classified as **anticoagulants** and

antiplatelet agents. The aim is to prevent formation of blood clots in the heart and aorta and in regions of vascular narrowing and irregularity. Brain ischemia is often caused by vascular occlusion, and blood clotting plays a crucial role in blocking the vessels. Of course giving an agent that will reduce the coagulability of the blood can potentially be disastrous if the stroke is due to hemorrhage. All antiplatelet and anticoagulant agents increase the risk of bleeding.

Antiplatelet agents mostly alter the function of blood platelets. When an artery becomes irregular and a plaque forms, the altered inner lining of the blood vessel stimulates platelets in the blood to stick to the surface of the plaque (adhesion) and to one another (agglutination). This creates a small white clot made of platelets and fibrin, which comes from fibrinogen, a serum protein present in the blood. The white clot subsequently can be displaced from the vessel and can embolize to vessels within the brain, causing TIAs and strokes. Platelet activation can also stimulate the formation of a superimposed red clot, made of red blood cells mixed with fibrin. One strategy to discourage platelet agglutination and adhesion is to give drugs that lessen these platelet functions. Some of the best-known examples of these antiplatelet agents are aspirin, clopidogrel, dipyridamole, and cilostazol. Sometimes the drugs are combined in one pill—for example, a combination of aspirin with extended-release dipyridamole. Most nonsteroidal drugs used for arthritis and pain relief also have some antiplatelet action; these drugs include ibuprofen and indomethacin. Some natural food substances such as omega-3 oils derived from fish, and black tree fungus (used in many Chinese dishes) are rich in substances that affect platelet functions.

One relatively new class of antiplatelet agents affects the attachment of platelets to fibrinogen. These drugs are called glycoprotein IIb/IIIa inhibitors. The most commonly used such drug is abciximab (ReoPro). It is given only intravenously in acute situations when white platelet–fibrin clots are thought to be blocking arteries.

Unfortunately, the use of these agents is sometimes accompanied by bleeding. Doctors are exploring other such drugs that can be given intravenously or by mouth.

Another strategy is to administer drugs that lessen the tendency for red clots to form, usually called **anticoagulants.** Although these drugs are often referred to as "blood thinners," they really do not change the thickness or viscosity of the blood; rather, they make the blood flowing in the vessels less likely to clot. A natural substance, **heparin,** or similar substances (heparinoids, low-molecular-weight heparin) are often given first by injection or intravenously while stroke patients are in the hospital; later, **warfarin**-type drugs (e.g., Coumadin) are given by mouth. Warfarin's activity depends on its influence on vitamin K, which is used by the liver to synthesize a protein called prothrombin that plays a vital part in the coagulation process. Prothrombin is catalyzed by activated factor X to make thrombin, which in turn catalyzes the reaction of fibrinogen to fibrin—a major component of clots.

To monitor the tendency for the blood to clot in patients taking warfarin-type anticoagulants, doctors order blood tests to compare the patient's tendency to clot against normal standards. The tests are called prothrombin time determinations and the results are given in time (e.g., 14 seconds), in a ratio of the patient's prothrombin time to local controls in that lab (e.g., two times control), or as a ratio determined by comparison with an international standard, the INR (international normalized ratio; e.g., 2.1 INR). The blood has to be monitored frequently at first to make sure that the results show enough lessening of clotting tendency without excessive risk of bleeding. Usually the physician, his or her nurse, or a laboratory will call the patient after the test and tell him or her how many pills to take that day and on subsequent days, and when to have the next blood test.

Blood coagulability and the effectiveness of warfarin are changed by many other drugs and by some foods. Warfarin dose is also affected by hormonal fluctuations in women (menstruation, pregnancy, ovulation, use of oral contraceptives, and female hormones used for any reason). Some of the factors that affect the dosage of coumadin and its effects are not known.

Newer anticoagulants are now being studied and introduced into medical care. Some agents (e.g., dabigatran and argatroban) have a direct effect on thrombin and do not work on prothrombin as warfarin does. Unlike warfarin compounds, the dosage of these **direct thrombin inhibitors** does not change and tests are not thought to be needed to monitor the extent of the effect on blood clotting. Dabigatran is taken as a pill twice a day. It was used to treat both Claire H. and Elaine S. to prevent the formation of new thrombi. Argatroban has to be given intravenously. Another group of agents act on factor X to prevent its conversion to activated factor X (Xa). **Factor Xa inhibitors** now available include apixaban and rivaroxaban. They are also less affected by foods and other pharmacological agents. Factor Xa inhibitors are given once or twice daily. Preliminary evidence from therapeutic trials indicates that these newer agents are as effective or more effective in reducing clot formation and cause less bleeding than warfarin. They may ultimately replace warfarin.

Neuroprotective Agents

Another treatment strategy to prevent or at least diminish brain ischemia is to give various drugs that reduce the vulnerability of the tissues to ischemia. These drugs are usually referred to as **neuroprotective agents.** In our earlier lawn analogy, their use can be likened to sprinkling something on the grass that would somehow make it more resistant to wilting in a drought. Neuroprotective agents or strategies can be given immediately after the first symptoms to patients with ischemia or threatened ischemia. The use of these drugs can give treating physicians a little more time to accomplish reperfusion and still preserve threatened brain tissue. One strategy being tested is cooling the body and brain below normal body temperature (hypothermia). This strategy has been used in the past during heart and brain surgery. When organs are at a lower than normal temperature, they require less energy. The theory is that the impaired blood supply will still provide enough energy to take care of the tissue's reduced demand.

Treating Acute Hemorrhage within or around the Brain

Compared to the complicated and multifaceted treatment of the different aspects of brain ischemia, treatment of bleeding inside of the head is more simple and direct. Aneurysms that cause sudden bleeding in the membranes that surround the brain (subarachnoid hemorrhage) can be clipped during surgery to prevent a second episode of bleeding. Aneurysms and vascular malformations can be obliterated by catheters placed within the feeding arteries through which various coils and other substances can be delivered to correct the abnormalities. Vascular malformations can also sometimes be removed surgically or can be destroyed by focused radiation. When brain hemorrhages are large and threaten life, doctors may be able to drain them by surgery. Reduction of blood pressure, and reversal of any tendency toward excess bleeding, can also be used to try to limit further bleeding into the brain.

Preventing Another Stroke

Prevention is always preferred to treatment after the fact. In Chapter 8, I reviewed various medical conditions and risk factors that predispose people to develop strokes. I also discussed primary prevention, meaning how to prevent strokes before they occur. The same principles also apply to preventing further strokes in patients who have already had one (secondary prevention). Here I emphasize some of the most important prevention strategies.

Controlling Hypertension

A variety of strategies are used to reduce elevated blood pressure. Losing weight and exercise are clearly quite effective in many patients. Reducing salt intake is also useful. A variety of different drugs are prescribed. Table 8-2 lists some classes of antihypertension drugs and the commonly used drugs in each class. Tom M.'s hypertension responded very well to labetalol, which was continued after he left the hospital. Often it becomes necessary to use more than one drug to control high blood pressure adequately.

Controlling Diabetes

Weight loss (in individuals who are overweight) and exercise are effective and important interventions for diabetic individuals. Diet is also very important; what you eat, how much, and when are all crucial. A variety of pills are used to reduce blood sugar; they are listed in Table 8-3. Patients who have very low levels of insulin are treated with injections of different types of insulin, sometimes more than once a day.

Lowering Blood Lipids

Reduction of high cholesterol and triglyceride levels is an important goal. This can be done in many patients by diet. In others, use of a statin (e.g., simvastatin, atorvastatin, pravastatin) is very effective in reducing total cholesterol levels. It has been shown that statins reduce plaque formation and stroke in patients who have arterial plaques and narrowing, even when their cholesterol levels are normal. Statins have a good effect on the lining of blood vessels in addition to their effect on blood cholesterol. The common drugs used to lower blood lipids are listed in Table 8.4.

Use of Anticoagulants and Antiplatelet Agents

Earlier in this chapter, I introduced the rationale for the use of these agents in the discussion of acute ischemic stroke. Both are also used in preventing first and subsequent strokes. Anticoagulants (warfarin compounds and direct thrombin and factor Xa inhibitors) have been used to prevent stroke in patients like Elaine S. who have atrial fibrillation. Antiplatelet agents have been shown to be very effective in stroke prevention in patients who have stroke risk factors, and in those individuals who have had a TIA or minor stroke.

Correcting Unhealthy Lifestyles

Smoking and heavy use of alcohol are well-established risk factors for stroke as well as other serious medical conditions. Stopping smoking is essential for anyone who has had a stroke or who has risk factors for stroke. One or two drinks of alcohol a day has not been shown to be harmful, but drinking more than that definitely poses a risk for stroke. Every effort should be made to have patients stop smoking and moderate their excess intake of alcohol. Other lifestyle changes, such as loss of excess weight and increase in physical activity, should be strongly encouraged.

Chapter 11

Complications

Strokes, like many other serious illnesses, can be followed by a host of other problems. I have often heard family members say, "Mom was okay when she got to the hospital with a stroke, but then complications set in." Complications are of three general types: (1) neurologic, causing brain function to worsen; (2) medical, involving organs other than the brain; and (3) psychological, as strokes are often followed by depression. Complications may occur during the hospitalization for acute stroke, or they can develop during rehabilitation and during later neurologic recovery.

Neurologic Complications

Worsening of Brain Ischemia

Despite the best medical treatment, the patient's brain function may deteriorate during the first hours and days in the hospital. Doctors characterize this worsening as "progressing stroke." Patients may enter the hospital with only minor symptoms, and then hours or days later develop quite severe loss of brain functions because of progression of their strokes. Minor weakness of the left arm and leg can progress to total paralysis of those limbs later.

The worsening is often due to continuation of the process that originally caused the stroke. For instance, in patients with hemorrhages, the bleeding can continue. Recall Tom M., the 61-year-old longshoreman with hypertension and a drinking problem who developed a hemorrhage into his brain. When he came to the hospital, he had a headache, felt very dizzy, and staggered when he walked. A CT scan showed that he had a hemorrhage in the cerebellum (see Figure 8-3). During the first hours in the hospital, his condition worsened and a repeat CT scan showed that the hemorrhage had grown larger. Patients who are hospitalized because of a subarachnoid hemorrhage due to a ruptured aneurysm may rebleed during the hospitalization before doctors can repair it.

Ischemic strokes are caused by an insufficient blood supply to a part of the brain. That insufficiency can persist and lead to a gradual or stepwise loss of brain function. For example, recall Robert H., the patient with an occlusion of a carotid artery in the neck. Such a clot can extend or embolize, causing further brain damage. In patients with brain embolism, the source of the embolus in the heart, aorta, or large artery, if not controlled, can throw off another embolus, causing further brain damage.

Brain Edema

Another important cause of worsening during the acute stroke period is brain edema and swelling. Injured tissue often induces a reaction around its perimeter that stimulates fluid to pour out of the tissue. Both brain hemorrhages and brain infarcts often become surrounded by an accumulation of fluid, referred to as brain edema. Think of an instance when you have struck an arm or a leg against something, creating a bruise. In the hours and days after the injury, the area around the bruised tissue often swells up. Edema often develops after a brain injury. The swollen tissue compresses nearby structures and is often accompanied by headache, worsening of the neurologic deficit, and a decrease in the level of alertness. Doctors can prescribe medicines to try to draw the fluid out of the brain.

Seizures

Seizures are not a very common complication of stroke but they do occur. In most patients the seizures that occur after strokes are relatively readily controlled with medicines. The brain is an electrical organ, made up of millions of nerve cells that transmit their messages electrically at synapses. Normally, the electrical activity of these cells is always related to activity in the environment and inside the body. A seizure can be thought of as a type of inappropriate activity or short circuit in part of the brain, during which some overactive nerve cells discharge spontaneously. These cells have been partially damaged by brain ischemia or hemorrhage, and they can discharge repeatedly even in the absence of an appropriate stimulus. A simple analogy is a failing lightbulb. Recall that sometimes when some of the lightbulb's filaments are worn out they will spontaneously light up for a moment and flicker uncontrollably even when the switch is turned off. Similarly, partially damaged nerve cells can discharge even when they are not stimulated.

Excessive discharge of local neurons can quickly spread through the nervous system, causing a seizure. Seizures take many forms. In some patients, they can be convulsive, during which there are violent contractions of the muscles of the limbs, face, and jaw. Often the muscles stiffen before they rhythmically jerk. Pelvic and abdominal muscle contractions during a seizure can cause a release of urine and bowel contents. Patients are unconscious during these seizures, and afterwards they usually do not recall the attack. In other patients the seizure spreads to both sides of the brain, and the patient looks blank and momentarily loses consciousness but does not shake. Sometimes the discharge remains local and patients develop localized jerking of muscles within their weak side. Sometimes the local discharge causes a visual, tactile, auditory, or olfactory experience, or an inappropriate emotional feeling. Sometimes the only obvious sign is cessation of speech or looking blank for a few moments.

When seizures complicate strokes, most often they develop after the acute stroke period when some nerve cells have partially recovered. The initial seizure(s) often can be very alarming to observers, even though patients are most often unaware of what happened during the seizure. Seizures are often followed by a period of drowsiness and decreased alertness; the nerve cells, having discharged vigorously, have used up a good deal of energy and require time to recover. Headache, tired and aching muscles, and a bitten tongue are also often present after motor seizures and indicate increased muscle activity during the seizure. Patients report their muscles feel as if they had been beaten up or as if they had run vigorously. At times after a seizure, patients can become temporarily violent and strike out at individuals who are trying to help them. Patients often recognize that they have had a seizure because of a gap in their recall of activities, or because of the feelings in their muscles, their sore or bitten tongue, and evidence of incontinence after they awaken.

Seizures almost always stop spontaneously. Observers need not stick anything in patients' mouths during a seizure. The idea that they can swallow their tongue is a myth. The seizing individual should be placed on a soft bed if possible, or at least in a place where they will not injure themselves during the shaking. If this is their first seizure, they should be taken to a hospital. When it is known that they are prone to seizures, they need not be taken to hospital afterwards unless the seizures are repetitive or if they don't wake up within 10 to 15 minutes. The treating doctor should be notified later so that medications can be adjusted when necessary.

Medical Complications

Pneumonia

Stroke patients often develop pneumonia in the hospital. A number of different factors related to stroke predispose them to the development of lung infection. Strokes often cause weakness of the structures within the mouth and throat that relate to swallowing food, liquids, and saliva. As a result, instead of proceeding from the mouth to the esophagus to the stomach, the swallowed substances can go into the larynx and from there into the lungs, which is called aspiration. Many different bacteria live in the mouth, and of course foods are not sterile. Infected material can thus reach the lungs and cause pneumonia.

Another factor that makes stroke patients susceptible to pneumonia relates to breathing functions after stroke. Individuals whose left arm and leg have become weak may also have some weakness of the left-side chest muscles that move air into the left lung. Especially in bed, the left lung is underventilated; it is much easier to take a deep breath if you are sitting or standing rather than lying flat in bed. Areas within the lung that are not well filled with air become more susceptible to infection. Stroke patients with weakness also may have difficulty coughing and clearing their airways of mucus and aspirated substances.

Doctors try and prevent pneumonia by not feeding by mouth stroke patients who have any difficulty swallowing. Encouraging patients to take deep breaths, and having them sit up in bed and breathe deeply, are other measures that help prevent the development of pneumonia. Early antibiotic treatment when pneumonia does develop is also important.

Urinary Tract Infection

Strokes often affect the mechanics of urination. Retention of urine and difficulty voluntarily emptying the bladder are common accompaniments of stroke. Passing urine is also more difficult in bed than when sitting at a toilet or, for men, standing. Compounding the urinary difficulty is the fact that most stroke-age men have enlarged prostrate glands and have had some difficulty in urinating even before their strokes. The tissues around the urinary passages in the pelvis are not sterile. When urine remains pooled in the bladder, infection very often develops. Bacterial infections within the urinary system can reach the kidneys and can enter the bloodstream.

Another common cause of urinary infections is the presence of an indwelling urinary catheter. Catheters are often inserted into the bladder of stroke patients who cannot urinate or who become incontinent. Bacteria have an easy entry into the bladder along these catheters. Intermittent catheterization is less likely to lead to urinary tract infection than leaving a catheter within the bladder.

Deep Vein Thrombosis and Pulmonary Embolism

Stroke patients are prone to develop **deep vein thrombosis** (DVT): blood clots within their legs, especially in limbs that are weak. These blood clots can travel to the lungs and cause pulmonary embolism, a life-threatening condition. Motion of the limbs, and contraction of muscles within that limb, keeps blood circulating in the veins. When stroke causes paralysis of the muscles in one lower extremity, and that leg is not moved normally after the stroke, the stasis of blood predisposes to clot formation. Many strokes cause activation of the blood clotting system, a factor that also predisposes to DVT.

A number of strategies are used to attempt to prevent clotting within the legs. Early walking and mobilization are important. Special stockings that help move blood along in the legs are also often used. Doctors also prescribe the anticoagulant heparin to patients who are not mobile; it is given in small doses by injection as a preventive anticlotting measure. Other anticoagulants described in Chapter 10 can be used instead of heparin.

Myocardial Infarction (Heart Attack)

Heart and brain vascular disease often coexist. Cardiac dysfunction is another frequent accompaniment of stroke. A dysfunctional heart may be the source of stroke, may coexist with stroke, or may be caused by the stroke. Many individuals who have disease of the arteries that supply the brain also have disease of the arteries that supply the heart; atherosclerosis is a condition that can affect many arteries. Heart attacks or atrial fibrillation can precede a stroke; in that case a clot has often formed within the left atrium or left ventricle of the heart and has embolized to the brain, causing the stroke. The preceding heart attack or atrial fibrillation may not have been diagnosed until after the stroke occurs.

In other patients the stroke precedes the heart attack. As I had mentioned during the discussion of DVT and pulmonary embolism, strokes can activate the body's coagulation system. This activation can cause clot formation to develop in already narrowed coronary arteries, leading to a heart attack.

Bedsores

Stroke patients with reduced mobility who can't reposition themselves and do not sense the need to change position are at risk of developing bedsores if they are not frequently turned and repositioned. Incontinence, by wetting the skin with an acidic fluid, increases the risk of developing skin breakdown. Prevention of skin ulceration is very important in stroke patients who have paralysis. Early mobilization is important. The skin should be kept clean and dry; stroke patients should be turned frequently. Adequate nutrition should be given. Pressure on arms and legs that have reduced sensation and on immobilized limbs must be avoided. The use of padded-heel boots can spare the heels from ulcers. Egg-crate mattresses, waterbeds, and soft cotton padding may help prevent the development of sacral pressure sores on or near the buttocks. Nurses often periodically check the entire surface of the skin, looking for any area of early breakdown. Particular attention should be paid to susceptible areas such as the buttocks, heels, elbows, wrists, between the toes, and the back of the head. If an ulcer develops, pressure on that area should be totally avoided, special mattresses should be used, and the wound should be dressed; if necessary, damaged tissue can be cut away to facilitate healing.

Contractures and Shoulder Pain

Immobility of the limbs, and maintenance in stationary, usually flexed positions can lead to fixed contractures at the knees and elbows. Decreased shoulder movement can result in shoulder pain, frozen shoulders, and swelling of the hand and forearm. When an arm is paralyzed, the weight of the limb hanging down can cause the upper arm bone (the humerus) to pop out of the shoulder joint. The weak arm should not be left to hang without support. Severe shoulder weakness and dislocation of the shoulder increase the likelihood of developing shoulder pain and swelling of the arm. Restoring full range of movement of the shoulder joint early is very important in preventing this unpleasant and disabling stroke complication. Physical therapists teach the patient and caregivers how to keep the shoulder mobile even when the arm is weak.

Osteoporosis

Studies of bone density after stroke show that there is a reduction in bone mineral density on the paralyzed side. Calcium removal from immobilized bone, lack of exposure to sunlight, poor nutrition with inadequate vitamin D stores in the body, and **osteoporosis** before the stroke increase the development or worsening of osteoporosis. It is most severe in those patients with severe paralysis, especially those who have prolonged immobilization. The reduced bone density predisposes to hip and other fractures, which tend to occur mostly on the paralyzed side. Early mobilization, exposure to sunlight, and giving calcium and vitamin D supplements can prevent or minimize this stroke complication.

Depression and Other Psychological Reactions

Patients' reactions to their strokes vary. New personality traits can emerge and old ones can become accentuated. Some patients see the stroke as a wake-up call. They fight vigorously to return to normal activities and pay more attention to their health and lifestyle than they did before their stroke. They view the stroke as a kind of blessing that awakened them to pursue better health. Others become angry at what they sense is an unfair punishment—"Why did God do this to me?" Like Job, they reason that they did nothing to deserve this handicap. Still others who had ignored their own risk factors feel guilty and upset at themselves for not being more health conscious and for not listening to their doctor. Many patients also feel guilty for placing a burden on their spouses and other caregivers.

Other stroke patients become depressed and feel hopeless about the future. One of the most important and yet most frequently overlooked complications of stroke is depression. Family members often report that Mom or Dad is no longer particularly weak and is able to get around well, but is not her or his usual self. Dependency and lack of social contacts are important factors in promoting depression. Patients who have a history of depression before their stroke are also likely to become depressed after a stroke. Studies show that the same medicines that help treat depression unrelated to stroke are also effective in stroke patients.

Chapter 12

What Are Some of the Dysfunctions, Disabilities, and Handicaps That Remain after a Stroke?

Strokes affect different portions of the brain and can lead to dysfunctions of many different types and severities. Chapter 7 describes the most common stroke symptoms, many of which are temporary. When symptoms persist and impair activities of daily living, they are often referred to as *dysfunctions* or *handicaps*. In this chapter I describe these different types of dysfunctions and disabilities, describing in depth those that are not especially familiar to most people.

Motor Abnormalities

The term *motor* refers to motion and movement of the limbs and body structures. Many patients become weak, stiff, or uncoordinated after a stroke. The severity of weakness varies from a very minor decrease in strength to paralysis—a total inability to voluntarily move a limb or a part of a limb. Most often weakness involves the arm, hand, leg, and foot on one side of the body. This pattern of one-sided weakness is referred to as hemiparesis (*paresis* means "weakness" and *hemi* refers to "half"); paralysis of the limbs on one side is *hemiplegia* (*plegia* means "paralysis").

> When one side is weak, hemiplegic patients find it useful to carry objects using an apron or hunting vest with multiple pockets.

The hand and arm are usually affected more than the leg and foot. The leg most often recovers enough to allow standing and walking, but hand recovery is usually not as complete. In other patients, only one limb might be affected. Sometimes the weakness involves the arms and legs on both sides of the body. (*quadriparesis* or *quadriplegia*).

When weak or paralyzed limbs begin to recover, they often become stiff, a condition referred to as spasticity. When doctors test the reflexes in spastic limbs, they are greatly exaggerated. Pressing a foot on the floor can lead to repetitive, jerky movements called clonus. Spasticity does have some benefit since support on a straight stiff leg is better than support on a leg that is loose and bends upon standing; weight bearing is difficult on a bent, weak leg.

Some patients' arms, legs, and gait become very uncoordinated after a stroke. Their hands and arms may shake when trying to pick up an object. Their walking can be very wobbly and off balance, like a person walking while drunk.

Motor disabilities also often involve the structures in the mouth and throat that are involved in speaking, handling food within the mouth, and swallowing. The lips, mouth, tongue, and throat are very active in speaking. Weakness of these structures often affects pronunciation of words and phrases. Speech can become lower in volume, slurred, and difficult to understand. Abnormal articulation of speech is referred to as dysarthria. Dysarthria must be separated from dysphasia, an abnormality of language, since the brain regions involved in production of language are very different from the motor regions that control the muscles of articulation. Very different conditions cause dysarthria and dysphasia.

Practicing speaking slowly, articulating each word, can make speech much easier to understand. Dysarthria is worsened by speaking rapidly.

Weakness of the larynx muscles makes the voice sound hoarse. Sometimes food gets caught in the throat, and the patient has to cough vigorously to get the food particles out. Most of the same muscles that control speaking are also involved in food manipulation within the mouth and throat and in swallowing. Difficulty swallowing is called dysphagia. Abnormal swallowing ability is a very important problem for stroke patients. Proper food and nutrition are key if patients are to repair injuries and maintain health. After a few days during which patients cannot swallow, a tube needs to be inserted either through their nose into the stomach (a nasogastric tube), or directly through the skin into the stomach (a percutaneous endoscopic gastrostomy), to maintain feeding and nutrition. Abnormal swallowing can also lead to aspiration: food particles, saliva, and bacteria from the mouth and teeth getting into the lungs instead going down the correct pathway into the esophagus and stomach. Aspiration often leads to pneumonia. Since some stroke patients have difficulty coughing and clearing their lungs and bronchial structures of sputum, pneumonia can be quite serious for them.

Because dysphagia poses such a risk, doctors are cautioned to evaluate swallowing ability in every stroke patient. Sometimes this is done by a bedside test of simply having the patient swallow water. At times special physical therapists will evaluate swallowing using X-ray techniques that can view and film materials as they are handled in the mouth, throat, and esophagus (video fluoroscopy).

Sensory Abnormalities

The term *sensory* refers to feeling on the limbs and body. Sensory abnormalities can include loss of feeling, abnormal sensations, or pain. Decreased feeling can involve the limbs, chest, and stomach on one side of the body. Some patients say that their sensory abnormality affects one whole side, as if a line had been drawn down their middle and everything on one side feels abnormal or less distinct. Loss of feeling often is present in the limbs that are weak.

At times the sensory abnormality is described as crossed, meaning it affects one side of the face and the other side of the body. The loss or decrease in feeling can be quite minor; for example, not being able to tell the difference between a nickel and a dime placed in the hand. In some patients, the loss of feeling can be severe so that they cannot feel any touch in an affected area. Loss of touch sensation is referred to as numbness or **anesthesia**. Sometimes touch is preserved, but patients cannot feel painful stimulation (**analgesia**). Often the involved limbs are insensitive to temperature; patients cannot feel hot, warm, cool, or cold on these limbs.

Instead of loss of sensation, sometimes the sensory abnormality comprises abnormal sensations that are described as tingling, prickling, pins and needles, burning, and the like. Patients often say that the region of abnormal sensation feels like a limb that "fell asleep" after being compressed for a while. These abnormal sensations are called paresthesias and can be quite annoying.

Sometimes painful sensations develop even in areas that are numb. Pain is usually not present in the early days and weeks after a stroke, but most often develops later. The pain can be described as an "icy cold pain," or as burning or sharp stabbing sensations. Painful feelings are often triggered by touch or use of the involved limb.

The body's sensory system can be simply thought of as having two different types of sensibilities. One type is related to coarse sensations such as pain and temperature sensations. Other sensations are fine and precise and relate to touch, joint position sense, and the ability to detect vibration on the skin and bony prominences. When all nerve pathways are intact, the finer sensibilities predominate. When these more precise sensory abilities are defective and parts of the body are anesthetic or show reduced fine-touch perception, then all stimuli seem to evoke only the coarse and unpleasant sensations described earlier.

I often explain the presence of pain by using an analogy with a radio. Suppose a radio is accidentally dropped into the water. At first, the radio does not work and no sound appears. When the wires dry out, sound returns, but moistening of the more delicate, fine radio wires impairs performance, and fine music is turned mostly into static. The louder the user turns up the radio's volume, the more the static will grate on the ears. Likewise, stimulation of an anesthetic limb stirs up unpleasant feelings that become more and more intolerable with increasing stimulation. Working with the arm during therapy and sleeping with unrecognized pressure on an arm can provoke severe pain. Unlike common pain that originates from local tissues, this pain is considered central because it involves abnormal function of nervous system tracts and does not indicate any local problem in the area in which the pain is felt.

Often explaining the nature of the pain to patients, and advising them to persist despite the pain, are helpful. Ordinary pain medicines are not very effective.

Cognitive and Behavioral Abnormalities

Thinking ability (cognition) is often affected by stroke. The nature of the intellectual change varies greatly. Loss of function can relate to the making of new memories, speaking, reading, writing, calculating, and recalling where things and places are located. There can also be many types of changes in personality and action.

Language Abnormalities

Proper language is extremely important for daily communication. Abnormal use and understanding of language is referred to as aphasia. Recall my description in Chapter 2 of the frustration that I felt when trying to obtain directions in Japan; the individuals I asked could not speak any English, and I couldn't speak, understand, or read Japanese. We simply could not communicate with each other despite the best efforts on both sides. This experience is probably similar to that felt daily by patients with severe aphasia.

One way to categorize the different types of aphasia is to divide abnormalities into motor (difficulty getting words out) and receptive (difficulty understanding what others say). In some patients with motor abnormalities, difficulty speaking can be slight and consist of using wrong or suboptimal words, but they can still get their meaning across to listeners. In others, speech difficulty can be very severe, rendering some aphasics completely mute or able to utter only syllables or repeat single words or phrases. Sometimes aphasic patients try to get meaning and emphasis across by varying the speed, emphasis, and loudness of their one word, such as, "fan...fan...fan" or "tan tan tan tan."

Patients with receptive aphasia have considerable difficulty understanding spoken speech. Some patients cannot understand speech at all. Unfortunately, most patients who have difficulty understanding what is said to them also have difficulty understanding written language, and so cannot read.

Some stroke patients lose the ability to read but retain the ability to speak normally and to understand spoken language. Alexia (difficulty reading) is often combined with loss of the ability to write and spell words normally. Loss of writing ability is referred to as agraphia. Some strokes make individuals suddenly illiterate—that is, they can no longer read, write, or spell correctly. Vision is handled in a different part of the brain than hearing (spoken language), so that alexia and aphasia can occur independently or together. Occasionally patients lose the ability to read, but retain the ability to write normally (alexia without agraphia).

Other types of communication relate to symbols; for example, musical symbols and arithmetic symbols. Some stroke patients lose the ability to interpret the meaning of these symbols. Stroke patients can become less adept at arithmetic; they may not understand the process of adding, subtracting, dividing, or they may understand the process but cannot get the answers correct. Lack of mathematical abilities is referred to as acalculia.

Loss of Memory (Amnesia)

Memory is a complex function that can be impaired in many ways by stroke. In one form of **amnesia,** stroke patients become unable to make new memories. They can hear and understand conversations and participate normally in activities, but 10 minutes later they will be unable to recall what was said or what they did. These amnesiac patients often repeat stories or conversations that they had just finished a few minutes before. They ask questions repeatedly even though the same questions have already been answered, sometimes many times. Repetitive questioning and hearing the same stories over and over can become quite tiring for caregivers and others who spend time with the patient. People become easily frustrated at repeating the same answers or conversation. In some patients, the inability to make new memories is temporary, lasting days, weeks, or up to 6 months. In others, loss of ability to make and retain new memories is permanent.

Strokes rarely cause a loss of old memories. Some people can vividly recall and describe events from their childhood and early married years, yet cannot recall what they did 15 minutes ago. Old memories are almost never wiped out by strokes.

Memory functions are represented on both sides of the brain within the cerebral hemispheres, but ideas, thoughts, names, and words are localized more on the left side of the brain, while visual memories are localized more on the right. When the left side is injured by stroke, patients may have difficulty remembering names; usually names of people are affected more than names of things. The inability to recall names is called **anomia**. The patient most often is unable to spontaneously recall the name, but they usually recognize the correct name when it is mentioned among others. When the right side of the brain is involved, their visual memory becomes defective. Such stroke patients may have difficulty recalling what things look like and remembering directions to and from various locations.

Abnormalities of the Amount and Timing of Activities

Some strokes affect patients' "get up and go." Their initiative declines, so that they are not motivated to initiate or participate in activities. They tend to sit and do little. Significant others describe them as "couch potatoes" or "bumps on a log." Unlike their previous behavior, their interest in others and in their environment seem greatly reduced. Some of these **abulic** patients can be stimulated by others to go out or attend a function with them, but when left to their own initiative, they seem content to just sit. These same patients also become less talkative. They seldom initiate conversations; when asked questions, their responses are short. They have difficulty continuing conversations or giving long, detailed replies. Some stroke patients cannot return to work because they have difficulty sustaining activity, even very simple, assembly-line-type work (which involves being able to continue to perform the same activity repeatedly and to persevere with the same functions).

The opposite situation may also develop after a stroke; that is, patients may become overactive and restless. They become easily agitated and can't seem to sit or lie still. They flit from one topic in a conversation to another and seem unable to maintain conversation, attention, or interest in any single subject or object. They exhaust themselves by overactivity. Sometimes these patients become so agitated that doctors call their behavior **delirium.**

Some patients are able to continue their usual functions but do so more slowly than before. Their speech is lower in volume and more often mumbled. They eat, speak, walk, and act more slowly, and it takes them longer to do activities than before their strokes.

Abnormalities of Planning, Judgment, and Performing Complex Activities

Some patients recover from their strokes, but do not seem to be able to function well in society despite what is seen as preserved intelligence and knowledge. In conversations their information level is the same as before their strokes. They have no limitations in performing single acts. When examined with the usual IQ tests they perform well, the same as before their stroke, yet their behavior and ability to act as they used to is severely impaired. Some categorize these types of abnormalities as executive dysfunctions, meaning that the patient has difficulty planning, organizing, and performing complex behaviors and functions.

To understand the nature of executive dysfunctions, it is important to review how unimpaired people decide whether or not to do something when presented with several alternatives. Let's look at the situation of deciding whether or not to move to a new apartment, and choosing among several possible apartments. Before acting, the careful, thoughtful individual will first examine the pluses and minuses of moving at all. What are the problems and good points of the present apartment: its size, condition, location, cost, upkeep, and the like? How does it fit with your present activities and responsibilities and those of your family: its proximity to jobs, schools, and shopping; safety and security; and other considerations? What would be better or worse about moving to another location? How do the possible new apartments stack up against the present apartment and against one other? Should you grab one of the other apartments now, or is it worth looking further because maybe a better apartment will come on the market?

This decision includes three different groups of behavior. The first is planning. Before acting, the person must thoughtfully weigh alternatives. Impulsive actions may not be in their best interest; inhibiting instinctive impulses is important. After deciding on an action, the person should plan how to carry it out, including considering the various possible situations that might arise (i.e., the what-ifs). The second is integrating various actions. To decide on the apartment, the person needs to assess and integrate multiple different types of information. This integration often means stopping one action and then beginning another, and then switching again to the first activity or another one. The last is judgment. To make a decision, the individual considers their own past experience, in addition to lots of environmental information. They then must weigh the options and ultimately make a decision.

Some stroke patients become unable to perform complex behaviors. An example is cooking a meal. First one must decide on what to include, considering many factors including health considerations, cost, availability, how things taste, and so forth. Then one must be sure to have all of the needed components. Often more than one part of the meal must be prepared at the same time as another. Otherwise, the food preparation might take all day, and some items would be cold when the meal is served. Some recipes require multiple actions and switching from one activity to another. Stroke patients with executive dysfunction simply cannot prepare a meal by themselves. These same people, however, can help with the preparation. They can perform individual tasks when someone else directs them. They just can't plan and integrate functions that are needed to get the meal together by themselves. They cannot multitask or adequately perform sequential actions.

Some stroke patients get stuck on a word or activity once started. They continue to repeat the same activity and response when they should move on to another query or behavior. This continuation is called perseveration, meaning that they persevere inappropriately with the same response or behavior. They cannot seem to change gears. Many complex activities require frequent switching from one activity to another and back again. For example when these patients asked to draw a square, they do so; but when asked to make a circle, they draw another square. They may stick out their tongue when asked to do so, but then protrude their tongue again when asked to raise their hands. They get stuck on the prior activity. They may also not be able to switch to a new topic of conversation, remaining mired in the last topic.

One stroke patient told me that he was afraid that his mind was seriously affected by his stroke despite the fact that all the IQ tests came out okay and he had no paralysis or other obvious disability. He was an executive in a large company. He customarily heard different presentations and proposals over the day, and before his stroke he was always able to arrive at a decision, choosing a proposal and then accepting or declining it. Now he found himself swayed by each proposal, feeling positive after hearing one presentation and then feeling just as positive about the next presentation, and finally not being able to choose between presentations. His ability to judge was compromised.

Some stroke patients become unable to inhibit instincts. They do not consider the effects of an impulsive act. One such patient after a stroke made a short list of everyone that he had always wanted to tell off: his fourth-grade teacher, minister, mother-in-law, and so forth. He proceeded to visit each one and tell them the criticisms that he had withheld before. Other patients become uninhibited about food intake, sex drives, or behavior. They act impulsively, giving in to instincts without considering the societal and personal outcomes of their behavior and its effect on others.

Difficulty Expressing and Interpreting Emotion and Feelings

As discussed in Chapter 2, speech can be divided into two different aspects: linguistic and affective. We have already discussed the linguistic part: the words themselves and what they mean. Loss of the ability to say words correctly and to understand their meaning is called aphasia. The other aspect of communicating with speech is affective. This includes all of the nonlinguistic emotions, moods, and feelings that accompany speech. By varying the volume, emphasis, facial expressions, cadence, and gestures that people use with their words, they can deliver very different messages. Abnormalities with the affective aspects of speech are often referred to as dysprosody, a word that literally means an abnormal speech rhythm. Depending on how a speaker says "Take the chair," the listener could conclude that she must take the chair or else their will be bad consequences, or it would be nice if she sat down but it is not required. Happiness, anger, fear, impatience, elation, despair, frustration, and other emotions and feelings are often transmitted along with our words. Reading a play and seeing the words is very different from seeing it performed on the stage by real actors.

Some stroke patients lose the ability to convey their emotions when they talk. They seem flat and unemotional. Some patients lose the ability to pick up the emotions and moods of those who talk to them. They fail to see that their spouses are upset, angry, or frustrated, and they do not detect body language signals. They lose the ability to tell when their spouse or significant other is tired and just does not want to talk and when they are eager to talk. People's wishes, feelings, and moods are typically obvious to those who know them from their facial expressions, voice, and bodily postures and gestures. Detecting body signals and moods is very important to living with and getting along with others. Losing the ability to convey or detect emotions and feelings is very disabling and disconcerting to those who live and interact regularly with the stroke patient.

Some stroke patients overexpress emotions. Most often these patients laugh excessively when things aren't that funny, or cry when things are not that sad. Sometimes they laugh or cry at inappropriate stimuli, such as laughing when the situation is sad. Most such patients have extensive motor abnormalities that especially affect speech and swallowing. The condition of overexpressing emotion this way is often referred to as pseudobulbar palsy, since it is most common in patients who have had multiple strokes that impaired the motor functions of muscles used to display emotions (those of the face, head, and neck). Patients with this abnormality are often quite sensitive about it and may avoid interacting with people because of it.

Visual Abnormalities

Looking and seeing are controlled by several parts of the brain. Looking is performed using areas of the brain that stimulate eye muscles to move. Seeing is of course done with the eyes, but the messages are transmitted to the brain through different pathways. Abnormal visual functions are very common after stroke. Since the eyes are supplied with blood by the carotid arteries, which also supply the cerebral hemispheres of the brain, blockage of these arteries can cause either temporary or persistent loss of vision in part or all of an eye. When the loss of vision involves a part of the eye, patients become aware of a hole (*scotoma*) in their vision in that eye.

When strokes affect the brain and not the eye, they most often involve structures that relate to vision on one side of visual space. Information from the left and right eye about objects and visual information on the right side of an individual is transmitted along pathways to the visual region located in the occipital lobe of the left cerebral hemisphere. When this pathway is damaged by stroke, patients become unable to see normally on their right side. This half-loss of vision is referred to as a hemianopia. Similarly, when the pathways in the right cerebral hemisphere are involved, patients lose the left side of vision. Some patients with a hemianopia are well aware that they can't see to the blind side, while others are unaware of the defect and bump into or miss objects on their blind side. At times, patients present to their doctors because of car accidents, bumping into parked cars, or objects that they could not see.

Drawing a red line along the far left of written pages can help patients with a left hemianopia to read. This line will help remind the reader to return to the line to catch the entire sentence.

The visual pathways that relate to the upper and lower regions of vision are also separated so that some patients lose only the upper or lower fourth (or quadrant) of their vision. Their visual defect is called a quadrantanopia. A man with a left upper quadrantanopia cannot see objects located in the upper part of his left visual field.

Some patients with strokes involving the right cerebral hemisphere develop a disorder referred to as neglect. They do not pay attention to objects or people located on their left side. They behave as if the left side of their world did not exist. Doctors sometimes test this by waving two hands directly in front of the patient, asking, "What do you see?" Patients with neglect always say they see only the hand on their right side.

Visual abnormalities related to stroke can involve complex visual functions that involve the relations of objects in space. Some stroke patients develop difficulty in recognizing people's faces, even ones they know well. They also may not be able to recognize familiar places or describe what objects or places look like. They cannot visualize in their mind's eye the appearance of objects, people, or places. They may not be able to describe where things are in their own rooms, houses, or neighborhoods. They may lose the ability to give directions for driving or locating places or to read maps. Patients may become lost even in familiar neighborhoods when they take a walk or drive a car. Artists may lose their ability to draw and copy. The size, proportions, and relationships of the objects in their drawings may become distorted and unnatural.

Some brain and motor abnormalities affect the movement of the eyes. Since the eyes usually work precisely together, when one eye does not work in full cooperation with the other, patients see double- two objects (diplopia). The objects may be alongside each other, directly above each other, or angled obliquely. Sometimes the objects seem to be moving or oscillating (oscillopsia) because the eyes themselves are jiggling and moving (nystagmus).

Urinary, Bowel, and Sexual Dysfunctions

Inability to control the bladder or bowels is often a very unpleasant experience after a stroke. Incontinence is embarrassing for the patient and often disturbing and upsetting to caregivers. Although everyone accepts the fact that babies cannot control their urine or bowels, somehow the same problem in adults is very difficult to tolerate, especially in our spouses, parents, and loved ones. Since sex involves the same anatomical regions, the potential of incontinence psychologically changes the sexual experience, introducing the possibility of soiling one's self or their partner during intercourse or other sexual activity.

The nerve centers that control urination, defecation, and sexual genital functions are located in an area of the lower spinal cord called the sacral region, which is comparable to the region in animals' spines that controls the tail. Many of its functions are reflexive. Filling of the bladder creates a sensation that signals the need to urinate, and filling of the bowel creates a sensation that stimulates bowel evacuation. Centers higher in the spinal cord and brain also control these functions.

Within the genital regions and anus are collections of muscle fibers called sphincters. When the sphincters contract, they hold in urine or feces. Relaxation of the sphincters by a message from the brain allows urine and feces to be expelled. When the urge to eliminate occurs, brain centers permit voluntary control over the sphincters until the person reaches a location where it is appropriate to urinate or move their bowels.

In patients who have had strokes, their control over urinary release is often affected and the reflex-induced bladder contractions are hyperactive, just as their limb reflexes can be exaggerated. As a result, once the urge occurs, they must quickly empty their bladders or risk being incontinent. Often they cannot control or feel the release of urine, especially when asleep. The voluntary control fibers are located on both sides of the brain. A stroke affecting one side of the brain, or the descending fibers on one side, usually causes only temporary loss of control over urination, since the other side will assume control with time.

At times the disorder of bladder and bowel function involves retention. Patients can become unable to urinate and require catheterization. This is very common in the days and weeks after a stroke, especially among older men who may have had some prostatic obstruction of their urinary passages before their stroke.

Similarly, brain centers control the anal sphincter. Normal adults can inhibit its relaxation until they reach a suitable place to defecate, but strokes can affect the ability to control bowel release, especially if the stools are loose. Bowel incontinence is a less common and less severe problem than urinary incontinence, since reflex functions are often sufficient to maintain bowel continence, especially with some training. Constipation is common in the early period after stroke, and can relate to inactivity and change in eating pattern.

Genital sexual functions also have local control centers in the sacral spinal cord and brain. Sexual instincts and activities are a important aspect of human existence over the entire life span. Sex is just as important and vital after 60 as during youth. Strokes can seriously impair sexual functions and inhibit normal sexual activities. The effects are multiple and include physiological, practical, and psychological factors.

The brain and the rest of the central nervous system control sex functions. The physiology of genital sexual-reflex functions, including erection, climax, and ejaculation in men, and clitoral erection and climax in women, is controlled in the sacral region—the same region that controls elimination. These functions can be temporarily lost or diminished after strokes, but are usually not permanently affected. The brain has more to do with desire for sex (libido) and for transmission of the desire for sex to the genital organs. Libido can be lessened or increased by strokes. In some patients, the same stimuli that produced sexual stimulation and interest before the stroke may not provide the same stimulation after the stroke. These physiological changes vary greatly depending on the location, type, and size of the stroke.

Psychological factors are also very important. Incontinence, and fear that a sexual partner might lose control of bowel or bladder function during sex, may subconsciously or consciously affect interest in having sex. Many spouses and sex partners are afraid that sex will precipitate a heart attack or stroke in their partner. Some caregivers see stroke patients (and patients who survive any serious illness) as somehow more fragile beings after recovery. Since sex can involve vigorous physical activity, caregivers are sometimes fearful that the patient will "break" in some unclear fashion. These caregivers are overprotective in every other way. Of course, some spouses were not very interested in sex even before their partner's stroke, and use the stroke as an excuse to decline sex. Some of the concerns and fears of the partners of stroke survivors can be allayed by open discussions; others are more irrational and can't easily be overcome directly.

Some patients are also fearful and psychologically unprepared to resume sexual activity. They often worry that their performance will prove wanting; as a result they will seem less of a man or less attractive as a woman to their partners. They are sometimes fearful that sex will precipitate another stroke, heart attack, or seizure, or injure them in some other way. Some of the fears can be allayed by simply trying and accomplishing sex, just as jumping in the water and swimming is the best way for children to overcome their fear of the water.

There are pragmatic practical barriers to sex also. Motor deficits may make positioning more complex, and mobility of the trunk and limbs can be reduced. Agility in attaining manual, oral, and genital stimulation may be affected. Loss of sensation in various regions after the stroke may diminish previously normal sexual arousal. Many stroke patients are able to resume normal or even heightened sexual activity after a stroke. When there's a will, there's a way.

Chapter 13

How Does Recovery from Stroke Occur? How Can Recovery Be Improved? What Is Rehabilitation? Where Is It Performed and by Whom?

Recovery

The great majority of stroke patients get better. Some improve so much that they return to normal or near-normal functions. Many are able to go back to their previous jobs and resume the same activities and interests that they had before their stroke.

There are three main mechanisms that explain improved function:

1. Some of the brain injury (ischemia, hemorrhage, and edema) can be reversible, and the tissue injury may be much less severe days, weeks, and months after the stroke than it was right after the event.
2. Very few if any brain functions are completely localized in one site. There are reserve regions that can perform similar functions; when one region is injured, other areas can take over. This process takes time and is clearly influenced by activity. For example, talking to and with aphasic patients clearly promotes the ability of uninjured brain regions to increase their language capabilities.
3. Adaptation to the deficits; that is, learning to do things in different ways than before.

The ability to return to normal function varies widely between individuals. Factors that relate to recovery of function can be divided into four groups: disease, anatomy, the person, and environment.

Disease-Related Factors

Hemorrhage and ischemia have different mechanisms, timing, and degrees of recovery. In patients with brain hemorrhages, the blood collects between brain regions, displacing but not often destroying normal tissues within the brain. Brain edema often surrounds the bleeding during the acute period after onset. Brain hemorrhages are gradually reabsorbed. White blood cells and other scavenger cells migrate to the region of bleeding. Chemicals are discharged, and very gradually the region of bleeding and brain edema dissolve and are reabsorbed, leaving a slit or hole in the brain in place of the blood. This slit disconnects functioning areas within the brain, but usually regions that surround the hemorrhage are preserved. Hemorrhages are associated with more mass effect than infarcts because extra matter (blood) is injected into the brain and skull.

Blood takes time to reabsorb. Recall when you have had a severe blow or fallen on an arm or leg, and developed a large bruise. The injury swells for a few days, and then the bruise heals very gradually over the following weeks—not right away. Similarly, patients with brain hemorrhages begin to recover later than patients with brain ischemia. The recovery period in hemorrhage patients is longer but recovery is often more complete than in patients with brain infarcts since usually less tissue is lost.

The process of recovery in patients with brain ischemia is quite different. The cause of the brain injury is lack of blood flow. In the minutes and hours after the symptoms begin, blood flow is often restored or at least improved. Emboli that have blocked an artery can spontaneously pass and move downstream. Even when main feeding arteries remain blocked, other blood vessels (collateral circulation) increase their contribution to the blood supply in the threatened region. The brain tissue receiving insufficient blood gives off chemicals that encourage ingrowth and expansion of blood vessels near the ischemic region. As discussed in Chapter 10, doctors can sometimes unblock the obstructed artery either mechanically (surgery, angioplasty/stenting, mechanical removal of clots) or by chemically dissolving the clot (thrombolysis). Improved blood flow allows recovery of some of the ischemic tissue.

When an artery is blocked, the tissue it feeds ceases to function normally, and patients develop symptoms that indicate loss of function. Within that undersupplied area there are different severities of injury. The area with the least blood flow, usually referred to as the **core** region, has the most severe injury and is almost always permanently damaged (i.e., infarcted). Areas beyond the core are often marginally deprived of blood; this tissue is often referred to as the penumbra. When blood supply to this penumbral area improves, the nerve cells in that region regain normal function. Since brain cells die quickly, the improvement in blood flow must develop within a few hours if they are to be saved.

Recovery of ischemic brain tissue can occur within hours or a few days if blood supply is improved. Sometimes the degree of recovery is dramatic. Patients with complete paralysis can recover complete use of their limbs; patients who are speechless can quickly begin to speak normally. However, infarcted tissue does not recover. Much of the recovery in patients with ischemia occurs within hours or a few days, in contrast to recovery of tissue in hemorrhages, which may take weeks to months. When a large portion of brain is infarcted, recovery is usually poor. In patients who have comparably sized hemorrhages and infarcts, more brain tissue is ultimately lost in the patients with brain infarcts.

Anatomy-Related Factors

As I have emphasized throughout this book, especially in Chapter 2, different parts of the brain have different functions. The location of the stroke is more important in determining the types of deficits and handicaps than the cause. For example, vision in the right visual field is located in the left occipital lobe. A hemorrhage or infarct in this region causes persistent loss of vision in the right visual field. By contrast, an infarct in the left temporal lobe could cause a severe loss of ability to make new memories. This amnesia almost always recovers during a period of 3 to 6, months even if the infarct remains unchanged. Memory abilities are located in both temporal lobes; injury to one causes only a temporary amnesia. Similarly, a stroke in the caudate nucleus on one side may cause temporary apathy that recovers even if the infarct does not. The location of the brain injury is an important determinant of recovery.

Many functions reside in more than one brain region. When one of these areas is damaged by stroke, other regions can allow substantial improvement of the lost function. When primary speech regions in the left brain are injured, other nearby regions in the left cerebral hemisphere, and some regions in the right cerebral hemisphere, can take over some of the lost language functions. Recovery by alternative brain regions is most common in children and young adults, but is possible at any age.

Some functions unfortunately are located predominantly in one brain region. Fine hand movements are controlled by the motor and sensory regions related to hand function (see Figure 2-8). When these areas are damaged by stroke, dexterity of hand function is lost and cannot be replaced by other brain regions.

The size of the stroke is also very important. Large infarcts and hemorrhages cause more persistent abnormalities than smaller ones. Recovery from large strokes is delayed and usually limited.

Personal Factors

We all recognize that some healthy individuals are motivated, well organized, determined, and successful, while others are often characterized using opposite adjectives. The attributes, capabilities,

education, training, and failings of individuals are even more important after a stroke, since they relate closely to the patient's ability
to overcome adversity. Individuals who have not been able to hold
a job before their stroke are extremely unlikely to be successful at
obtaining and keeping a job after it.

Prior health conditions are also very important. Recovery from
a paralysis of one side of the body (hemiparesis) requires considerable determination, work, and stamina. Patients who have arthritis
or prior injuries of their lower limbs have more difficulty learning to
walk well than those who had strong joints and limbs before their
strokes. Prior heart and lung disease, being overweight, or being out
of condition of course also affect individuals' ability to generate the
stamina needed for rehabilitation efforts. Depression, which is very
common after strokes, likewise affects the will to recover.

Determination and personal strengths and abilities weigh heavily on recovery. "When the going gets tough, the tough get going"
is an old saying that applies well to stroke recovery. Various people
recover quite differently from the very same type, location, and size
of stroke.

Environment-Related Factors

Personal, interpersonal, social, and economic resources are extremely
important for stroke recovery. The most important resource is the
presence of one or more significant others who will give the stroke
patient quality time, physical help, emotional support, and encour-
agement. When you have a handicap, it is extremely hard to go it
alone. Such ordinary considerations as having the use of a car, living
on one floor (especially the first floor), the presence of an elevator
in an apartment building when the patient lives on an upper floor,
accessible shopping, and handicap precautions and facilities can
make a great deal of difference in determining what stroke patients
will be able to do and accomplish. Economic resources to pay for
adequate equipment and help are also very important.

Adaptation to the home setting is a major focus of rehabilitation. The home often has to be changed a bit to adapt to the handicaps of the stroke patient. Placing grab bars in the shower and bath, discarding throw rugs that could result in tripping or falls, and building ramps for ready entry into the home are examples of the modifications that are sometimes needed.

Rehabilitation Hospitals and Wards

Recovery is a word that describes the process of getting better. The focus is on the person or group that has been injured, or in this case the individual who has had a stroke. The term **rehabilitation** has a different focus; it refers to the process of others helping to promote recovery. Rehabilitation can take place in a special ward or hospital, at an outpatient facility, or at home. The choice of location depends heavily on the nature and severity of the disabilities and handicaps that are present after the stroke, and the facilities and personnel available in the community and at home.

Rehabilitation can be offered at rehabilitation hospitals, subacute nursing facilities (SNFs), or at home. The location is often dictated by insurance carriers; unfortunately, "he who pays the piper often calls the tune." There are many differences between these sites. Hospitals usually have doctors available 24 hours a day, laboratory and radiology services, and a range of available physician consultants. Therapies are usually offered 3–4 hours a day, 6 or 7 days a week. Physician availability is much less at SNFs, and therapies are usually performed only 2–3 hours a day, 5 days a week. Laboratory facilities are usually lacking. Outpatient and home therapies have the advantage of allowing attention to adaptation to the patient's actual environment, but they are limited to those individuals who have relatively minor handicaps that can be managed at home.

The personnel, aims, and functions at rehabilitation hospitals are quite different from those found in acute-care hospitals.

In an acute-care hospital, the prevailing strategy is to diagnose and treat medical illnesses. By contrast, the goal of rehabilitation is to correct and adapt to various handicaps in order to maximize functions. Of course, some rehabilitation and physical therapies should have been started during the stay at the acute-care hospital. Medical care begun at the acute-care facility should be continued during rehabilitation.

The first step toward remediation of and adaptation to disabilities is an accurate assessment of what the patient can and cannot do. Testing is often accomplished by a series of different people that might include physicians; nurses; psychologists; physical, speech, and occupational therapists; and social workers. The doctors are often physiatrists (also called physical medicine specialists) rather than neurologists. Sometimes internal medicine specialists, geriatricians, and neurologists are active in rehabilitation centers or available for consultation. The doctors who provided care at the acute-care hospital are rarely available during rehabilitation unless it takes place in a ward or other building located near the facility where acute care was given.

One of the major characteristics of rehabilitation hospitals is their emphasis on a team approach, with a number of different individuals working together to characterize deficits and enhance recovery of functions. Each usually begins by testing different functions. Speech therapists may test language and swallowing functions if abnormalities are suspected. Physical therapists test the strength and agility of the arms and legs and watch the stroke patient walk. Occupational therapists determine if the patient can perform various common tasks of ordinary daily living and working. Neuropsychologists test thinking functions such as memory, language, perseverance, and visual-spatial abilities. Social workers explore the patient's family, community, and financial situations and resources so that care can be continued after. Physicians review medical aspects, including past and present medical illnesses, and the cause and treatment of the stroke.

Once testing is completed, there usually is a group meeting in which the patient is fully discussed and plans of management are agreed upon. Each person who will be involved in therapy then actively tries to help the patient overcome their deficits. Staff meetings are regularly and frequently held to discuss progress.

For a stroke patient to overcome a deficit, it is very helpful if he or she recognizes exactly what is wrong. That is the first step toward recovery. Education about the nature of the potential handicap is very important. For example, many individuals who have a visual field abnormality do not recognize or understand that the problem is not in the eye, and do not realize what they are not seeing. Let's consider Robert H., a patient with a left visual field defect who had difficulty attending to and seeing objects to his left. Showing him that he wasn't noticing objects or words on his left and that he did not look towards the left was the initial step toward retraining his visual focus. Such a patient is trained to always look toward the blind side and to make sure that they have gazed to the far outer edges of reading material, pictures, and scenes, lest they miss objects and people on their blind side. The education process should include the caregivers who will be with the patient when he or she returns home.

Different therapists tackle various types of deficits. A physical therapist may work on limb strength and exercises and walking stability. They may help train patients with paralysis in transferring between bed, chairs, and the toilet. When the patient has a weak arm or leg, the therapist will show him or her how to improve its function. They may teach patients how to stretch stiff limbs, and also show caregivers how to perform range-of-movement stretching procedures that should be continued once the patient goes home. Physical therapists also may show the patient how to use canes, walkers, and similar aids.

Occupational therapists may work with a patient in a makeshift kitchen to help them resume cooking functions. They will review with the patient how to perform various daily activities. They also may collaborate with the caregivers to help adapt the home according to the stroke patient's specific handicaps and disabilities.

Speech therapists may concentrate on the patient's speaking, reading, and writing skills and may also evaluate and treat swallowing problems. A number of computer programs are now available to help patients with aphasia. The speech therapist will often begin courses of speech remediation that will be continued in an outpatient setting after discharge from the rehabilitation hospital. They also may work with the caregiver to determine the best way to manage the patient's speech difficulty at home.

Rehabilitation hospitals also usually have individuals who can make and fit various devices such as braces, slings, and supports that can help patients perform various functions. The strategies are to correct the functions that can be corrected, but also to find alternate means of doing things that cannot be readily corrected. For example, a right-handed person who develops paralysis of the right hand will be taught to do things more often with the left hand. When an individual cannot use their hands to grasp small objects, various aids are used to facilitate hand functions.

The process of recovery usually takes much longer than the time it takes to develop the stroke. Stays in the rehabilitation hospital are usually longer than stays in the acute-care hospital. Much of the patient's recovery is spontaneous and related to the injured brain area recovering and other regions taking over lost functions. As mentioned, many functions are represented in more than one place in the brain. If one area is injured, other regions can assume the lost functions with time and training. This is especially apt to happen in children.

A very important aspect of the rehabilitation process is to educate significant others in the patient's home and environment about the nature of the various handicaps and how they should be handled when the patient returns home. Wives, husbands, children, other family members, and lovers can help with the therapy and should know the patient's abilities and limitations.

The stay in a rehabilitation hospital may not succeed if the patient has very severe disabilities. If the patient cannot go home, they are often transferred to a SNF for continuing but less intensive therapy. The timing of the transfer often depends on insurance coverage. The rehabilitation hospital staff may readjust the recovery goals for the patient; for example, improving mobility enough that the stroke patient can be easily assisted, rather than aiming at independence.

When patients are ready to leave rehabilitation hospitals or SNFs, it is very important that discharge planning is performed to guide further recovery strategies and outpatient therapy if needed. Outpatient therapy can help considerably by supervising therapies aimed at restoring strength, balance in walking, and fitness.

Outpatient Therapy

Some patients are discharged home after their stay in the acute hospital. They are often referred for outpatient therapy either at home or at an outpatient facility. Other patients continue outpatient therapy after leaving a rehabilitation facility.

1. The caregivers should view therapy sessions and be instructed by the therapists in the techniques used. The caregivers then can supervise and promote therapy between outpatient visits.
2. Patients recovering from stroke should practice the techniques learned during the therapy sessions between therapist's visits. Stretching and exercise are very important and should be done daily.
3. Rest periods are important. Rest can be alternated with exercise and activity.
4. Therapy in the home and in the workplace is particularly useful, since the recovering patient can learn to use and work with their usual objects and perform their former routines.

5. After the patient stops regular therapy, it is helpful for their therapists to conduct periodic reviews to ensure that the patient is not developing new bad habits and is continuing to follow instructions given during the initial therapy period.

Rehabilitation and Exercising Can Be Overdone

It is very important to emphasize that much of the recovery from stroke is natural. The stroke damage heals, and nature finds a way to restore some of the compromised functions. Recovery goes on via the determination of the stroke patient and their caregivers and significant others—without continuing formal rehabilitation. One problem that I find very often in relation to rehabilitation and therapy is an intense attachment of the stroke patient to therapy and their therapists. Most physical and occupational therapists are young, active, encouraging individuals who work closely with patients. Because the patient improves while they are having therapy, many patients automatically associate recovery with therapy and worry that they will regress or stop improving when formal therapy is stopped. Recall that therapy occurs during the period when natural recovery is maximal. Many patients who do not have formal therapy do get better. There comes a time when patients should stop going to formal therapy. After all, therapy takes time and effort, and most patients must travel to the therapy location. There comes a time when they must return to living as a person— not as a patient.

There is another issue that relates to the aim of therapy and the specific therapies used. Because therapy often targets very specific functions (e.g., arm and hand strength and dexterity), patients will continue to vigorously work at those exercises—in this case, arm- and hand-strengthening maneuvers—firmly wedding in their minds recovery from stroke to the return of these upper-limb activities. But the aim of rehabilitation is not to return all functions to normal. That is an impossible goal. The aim is to return the individual stroke patient to *as normal daily living as possible*. Patients without normal hand function on one side can live quite normally and do most everything they could do before. There have been baseball pitchers and successful politicians who have only one functioning arm. Patients should be encouraged to broaden their view of recovery toward resuming normal activities. Overemphasis on therapy and special exercises delays the return to normal functioning and socialization. The individual who has had a stroke must resume thinking of themselves as a person, not just as a sick receiver of care—a patient. Life is short. Try to gain as much as you can from each day. Time spent on therapy and exercises is lost for other activities that you might enjoy, such as movies, travel, reading, or just schmoozing with friends and family.

Chapter 14

How Does One Person's Stroke
Affect Others?

"It takes a village to raise a child."

—HILLARY CLINTON

If a village of folks is needed to adequately manage a child, it takes several villages to care adequately for a stroke patient. Strokes don't just happen to individuals. Although only one person has the stroke, the effect of that stroke is quite widespread. The family constellation and members' roles often change. The spouse or significant other now must become a caregiver in addition to previous roles and responsibilities. Children and grandchildren are affected. The stroke patient's role at his or her workplace may end or be altered. Community and religious organizational activities are likely to change. The physical, social, psychological, and economic burden is enormous.

The Caregiver

Surveys and research have now begun to collect information from caregivers about their activities and stress levels. Most caregivers are husbands and wives. They are usually around the same age as the stroke patient. They often have similar health problems and their own ills and handicaps. Their former relationship with their spouse may be drastically altered by stroke. If the caregiver is a woman (which is more likely), she may have been the more passive individual in the household, and the stroke patient may have been the more dominant figure and the decision maker. Now, as the caregiver, she must call the shots and take the lead in decisions, an unaccustomed role that may make her feel ill equipped and rather uncomfortable. On the other hand, a male caregiver may be very unaccustomed to dealing with house-related day-to-day issues that his spouse had always handled. Multiple new roles, all new, place enormous stress on the caregiver and on interpersonal relationships with the stroke patient.

Nurse

The stroke patient may require activities that nurses or nursing assistants usually perform in the hospital. These may include supervision of medications and even sometimes injecting medicines like insulin and low-molecular-weight heparin after appropriate training. Attention to toileting and incontinence are especially stressful for some caregivers. The caregiver often learns to ask about feelings, needs, discomfort, new symptoms, and other unfamiliar areas. Most caregivers have had no training in these nursing activities.

Amateur Psychologist/Cheerleader

Depression is very common after stroke. Studies show that having a significant other to encourage, lead, push, and cajole the patient is the single most important factor in their return to the workplace and to former roles in the family and community. The caregiver must remain upbeat. And yet the additional roles and stresses often lead to discouragement and depression in the caregiver. He or she must remain positive in the face of increased responsibility, role reversals, and stress.

At times, the stresses on caregivers become so great that they selfishly choose to bail out of their relationships and responsibilities.

Despite the fact that the marriage vows say "in sickness and in health," illness and time often change loved ones from the person that they married to a totally different individual. Some significant others and family members simply cannot cope with the change, the stresses, the responsibilities, and the change in attention from the *me* to the *you*.

Therapist/Trainer

In patients with residual physical handicaps, the caregiver often assumes roles that physical, occupational, and speech therapists carry out in rehabilitation facilities. During rehabilitation, the caregiver should be shown the exercises and activities that need to be practiced and performed when the patient returns home. This often includes how to shift from bed to chair, how to stand, beginning to walk, maintaining gait, getting on and off toilet seats, use of eating utensils, and so forth. Caregivers frequently need to carry out exercises through the patient's full range of movement to keep their limbs from stiffening. They may also require training in supervising the stroke patient's bathing and toileting.

Amateur Physician

Before and during the stroke and its recovery, the patient and caregiver are likely to be exposed to many health professionals. Their primary care doctor or internist, the neurologist involved during the acute-care hospitalization, and the rehabilitation personnel may all be different people. Unfortunately, medical information about the stroke and its cause and management may not have been communicated as thoroughly as possible to the patient's primary care physician, who was likely not to have been involved during the acute hospitalization and rehabilitation. Also, surveys have shown that many primary care doctors and internists are not up to date on the diagnosis and treatment of stroke and its complications.

Of course, most caregivers are untrained medically. Brain functions and abnormalities are complicated to understand, and many people either have not been taught effectively, or have been taught and still cannot grasp the information about the brain, stroke, and various handicaps. They often do not know what to expect, what to look out for, or whom to call. The situation is much like a first-time mother who has no training or experience in handling a tiny, helpless being who can't communicate effectively.

Pharmacist

Nowadays when I ask patients in my office to show me what medicines they take, they often unload a bag full of bottles—often more than 10. How can anyone keep all of these pills straight? Sometimes I find that two of the bottles contain the same substance, one under the drug's brand name and the other under its generic name. Questions about the pills abound. When is the best time to take them? Which ones should not be taken together? Which need to be taken with food? Which require patients not to eat for a period of time after use (e.g., some osteoporosis pills)? Which over-the-counter drugs (e.g., for pain, colds, or insomnia) should not be taken because of illnesses or because they react badly with the patient's medicines? The use of medicines can be complex, and the patient's doctor or pharmacist may not easily be able to answer all of these questions, especially if they come up after hours.

Pill boxes that are preloaded for the week and by time of day are very helpful, but filling them may be beyond the ability of many caregivers to perform without help.

Banker/Economist

Strokes clearly cost money. Salaries and other money that the stroke patient earns may diminish, despite any disability insurance. The caregiver also may have to curtail some of their work.

Medicines, transportation, and doctor visits all cost money. The bills may add up. Many caregivers, especially women, have not had previous experience with handling the family's money, bills, or investments of the family.

Spouse/Companion/Lover

The caregiver will want to continue their accustomed role with the stroke patient, but the new responsibilities and stresses may make this very difficult. I commented in Chapter 12 on changes in sex function after stroke. Decreased erectile function is common in men, and reduced sexual urges and responsiveness are common in both sexes. Other handicaps such as weakness, difficulty manipulating the body and limbs, and incontinence, can affect the ability to perform sexual acts and functions.

Personality and behavioral changes in the stroke patient also may alter interpersonal relations. Some stroke patients develop a lack of initiative and apathy; lethargy; aggressiveness; difficulty picking up body language, vocal tone, and facial expressions; difficulty speaking; depression; and other previously unaccustomed traits that alter the relationship between the stroke patient and the caregiver.

Multiple Caregivers

The previous discussion assumes that one individual will assume the role of direct caregiver, usually when the stroke patient returns home. Sometimes there are more than one caregiver. This occurs most often when the stroke patient has to go to a nursing home or other chronic care facility. The task for the spouse or significant other, if there is one, is to try to monitor the staff's delivery of care, hoping that it will be done with attention, kindness, and concern for the health and welfare of the patient. Care assessment is difficult at best; it usually means traveling to and from the facility at frequent intervals to render care.

Sometimes the responsibility of caregiving is shared among family and friends. The challenge here is to divide up responsibilities and caring evenly and fairly, and for all of the caregivers to have similar goals. This task often causes stresses on relationships that had been tenuous before the stroke. Often the participants have other major demands on their time and effort.

Children and Grandchildren

Children of stroke patients are, by nature, accustomed to a dependent relationship with their father or mother. Now an adolescent or young adult child may be thrust into a different role with their parent. In a book I wrote with a colleague, *Striking Back at Stroke: A Doctor-Patient Journal*, the patient's oldest daughter reflected on the changes in her life that her mother's stroke produced. She became a caregiver. She described the strain of added responsibilities and the lack of parental guidance. The usual dependency role between parent and child had been abruptly reversed and was difficult to recapture. Doctors and nurses should emphasize to caregivers that they may need to pay even more attention to their children after a spouse's stroke. Those of us who have children know that bringing a new baby brother or sister home to a child is a big stressor, and that extra attention must be given to that child. The family must be kept together, and spirits should be upbeat to meet the challenge. Everyone must pull together to meet the new challenges while continuing previous roles and responsibilities.

Relationships with Grandma and Grandpa are often very special for children. A special bond may exist. Grandchildren are often devastated by the occurrence of stroke or other disabling illness in a beloved grandparent. They, too, may need extra attention and explanations during the recovery period and thereafter. Often the illness or death of a grandparent is a child's first encounter with serious loss.

The Workplace and the Community

Many stroke patients had worked for long years in one job or for one company. The sudden absence of that individual affects the workplace. Return to work is often possible, but sometimes the tasks and responsibilities performed before the stroke cannot be continued. The flexibility at the workplace may be limited, so that a change in job description that meets the stroke patient's capabilities may not be possible. Also, a new job might be very difficult to acquire.

Chapter 15

What Does the Future Hold?

"It is difficult to make predictions, especially about the future"
—YOGI BERRA

I do not have a magic crystal ball that can accurately predict the future. Perhaps what I will share in this chapter are my own hopes, wishes, and dreams rather than predictions. Since the development of a proven treatment for stroke, thrombolysis, stroke seems to have come of age. The U.S. government, the media, the American Academy of Neurology, the American Neurological Association, the European Stroke Organization, the American Heart Association, and the American Stroke Association have all pressed for more research and more availability of expert care for stroke patients. Clearly there will continue to be important advances in our knowledge about the various causes of stroke and about treatment.

Education of Doctors and the Public

Doctors cannot treat stroke patients optimally unless they come to medical facilities soon after the onset of stroke symptoms. For patients to come early, they must be aware of stroke and its manifestations. Yet numerous surveys have shown that the public's knowledge about stroke is very limited when compared to its awareness about heart disease and cancer. One of the reasons for this lack is its complexity. The brain is much more diverse and complex than the heart. Understanding the symptoms of stroke and its effects on individuals requires some knowledge of brain function. The symptoms and signs of cancer and heart disease are much simpler and more homogeneous that those of stroke.

The process of biology and health education is critical and must begin early, in schools. Our children must be taught more about their bodies and their natural functions than previous generations. Science and mathematics education in the United States is weak compared with Europe and some parts of Asia. We need more money and support for public education. More health education and information also should be provided in the workplace, in the media, on the Internet, and through doctors' offices and hospitals.

The education process should extend also to primary care doctors, internists, and emergency physicians. Advances in medicine and technology come so quickly that it has been very difficult for physicians to keep up. Sadly, most generalists are not particularly knowledgeable about the brain and stroke.

Technology

Technology is now available that can show the brain and its blood vessel supply quickly and safely. I have described the diagnostic technology now used in Chapter 9. Improvements in technology have occurred so rapidly during the last decade that I can reliably predict still further improvement in the near future. However, many facilities that care for stroke patients do not have readily available modern imaging technology. In the future, more centers will have modern CT and MRI capabilities.

Ultrasound technology has improved even more than other brain imaging. Ultrasound also has important advantages over CT and MRI. Diagnostic ultrasound equipment is much less expensive. It is portable and can be brought to patients in emergency rooms, outpatient facilities, and hospital wards. Ultrasound testing can be repeated often, and the cost to the patient is relatively low compared to CT and MRI. In some European medical centers, neurology trainees are taught to use ultrasound probes so that testing can be done as part of the initial evaluation by the doctors when they examine the patient. Perhaps in the future, ultrasound and even CT scanning might become available in ambulances and be performed in the field when the patients are first seen. I hope and believe that the use of ultrasound will continue to spread to medical centers and stroke units that now do not rely extensively on ultrasound results.

Devices used for treatment have also advanced, and much new technology is available for trying to open blocked arteries and treat aneurysms and vascular malformations. Newer catheters, clot-removing devices, and removable stents recently have been introduced into stroke treatment and medical trials. Advances undoubtedly will continue in the technical equipment used to treat a variety of stroke conditions.

Stroke Centers

Until recently, any hospital could advertise as a stroke center. If they were objectively evaluated, however, many of these self-designated stroke centers would not qualify as such. Accurate diagnosis and treatment requires that specialized stroke centers have expert stroke care readily available 24 hours a day and 7 days a week. This capability requires doctors experienced in stroke and systems in place to ensure that stroke patients are handled quickly and effectively. Centers specializing in stroke also have the technology available to diagnose the type and location of stroke and the physicians experienced in interpreting the tests. Testing can and should be done quickly. Not many hospitals live up to these requirements, but most large cities have stroke centers at one or more hospitals.

Many federal and state governments have established rules for designating stroke centers. Hospitals must apply for the designation; evaluators then check the hospitals' capabilities and approve or deny the application. Primary stroke centers have adequate personnel and technology, but may not have the most advanced services, while other centers will be designated advanced centers because they have complete medical and surgical capabilities, up-to-date technology, and effective protocols that ensure rapid and efficient throughput of patients suspected of having stroke. The number of qualified designated stroke centers will no doubt increase during the near future.

Stroke Specialists, Stroke Units, and Communication Between Physicians

This book should have already convinced readers that stroke is a very complex and diverse condition. The brain is complicated, and so are the many diseases that involve the brain, including stroke. Advances in knowledge, technology, and treatment have come so quickly that it has become almost impossible for general physicians to keep up with modern stroke evaluation and treatment. Clearly more stroke specialists are needed and without a doubt will be trained to meet the demand.

Most stroke centers are specialized, self-contained areas within the hospital called stroke units. The nurses and doctors in these units have a special interest in stroke and are trained and experienced in caring for stroke patients. The physician in charge of the unit is most often a stroke specialist. A team that usually includes doctors, nurses, therapists, and social workers treats and consults about stroke patients within the unit. Stroke units have proliferated in Europe and have been shown to reduce mortality, decrease the number of patients who go to chronic-care facilities, increase the number of patients who go home, and reduce long-term disability and the cost of care. It is widely agreed that stroke units improve the care of stroke patients, and more hospitals will develop stroke units in the future.

In most regions of the United States, the care of stroke patients is divided among several caregivers. Acute treatment is rendered at hospitals, often by hospitalists and full-time staff physicians.

Rehabilitation and recovery often occur at other hospitals that are staffed by different physician specialists and care teams. After the patient returns to the community, primary care physicians are entrusted with follow-up and secondary prevention. These same community physicians may have cared for the patient before the stroke and were involved with primary prevention and the general care of the patient. Communication among professional caregivers is often suboptimal—one hand doesn't know what the other has done or is doing. Systems need to be improved; through new computer technology (and old-fashioned but still useful phone calls), communication between caregivers will become more efficient.

Connecting Patients to Stroke Centers

Two important problems will need to be addressed in the future. The first is how to deliver potential stroke patients living in large urban areas quickly to one of the most advanced stroke centers in that city. In many areas of the country, ambulance personnel are instructed to bring every urgent patient to the nearest hospital, regardless of its stroke capabilities. By contrast, government rules instruct ambulances to bring patients with serious trauma to the nearest qualified and designated trauma center. Similar regulations are needed for stroke. Patients should be delivered urgently to the nearest advanced stroke center. In many European cities these regulations and practices already exist. Patients and governmental bodies need to become aware of and disseminate information about stroke centers and their qualifications.

The second major issue relates to patients in rural communities where there are no stroke centers. How can rural and suburban hospitals connect with stroke centers to optimize treatment? One predictable development will be an increase in so-called telemedicine. Using telemedicine, hospitals can connect via computer technology to one or more other medical centers, allowing doctors at one hospital to consult with experts at another. Some regions of Europe and America have arranged hub-and-spoke relationships: peripheral spoke centers communicate with one hub center that furnishes 24/7 coverage. Computer facilities allow an image of the patient to be transmitted along with results of diagnostic tests. This lets doctors at the referral center interview the patient, observe and at times direct the examination, and view the available brain and vascular images. In this way, rural hospitals and non-specialized stroke centers can consult quickly with physicians at stroke centers for guidance. Should the patient be transferred to a stroke center? By ambulance or helicopter? What further testing is required? What treatments should be given? At the receiving stroke center or after infusion of an agent ("drip and ship")? Thus management of the patient can be shared between the local physicians and the stroke center. Use of telemedicine will undoubtedly spread during the next decades.

Newer Treatments and Refinement of Existing Treatments

Modern stroke treatment is really in its adolescence. Some drugs only recently have been introduced, and doctors and patients are still learning about the effectiveness and safety of these substances. New drugs are being developed and tried every year. Devices have also proliferated; they vary widely and now include stents for opening arteries and keeping them open, retrieval devices for removing emboli from arteries, devices for closing holes within the heart and preventing heart arrhythmias, and various filters for preventing emboli from the heart and arteries from reaching the brain and other organs during procedures. In the future, even more devices and drugs will be developed and brought into clinical practice.

Emphasis on Recovery after Strokes

During the past decade, the emphasis has been placed on prevention of stroke and on acute, urgent treatment of patients with stroke during the first few hours after the onset of symptoms. This has been very important since it has brought stroke treatment to the forefront of public attention. Unfortunately, this approach will never completely solve the problem. Most patients do not arrive at medical centers that are well equipped to manage acute stroke in time for urgent treatment. Even when treatment is given in time, residual neurologic signs often remain. The result is that many patients will survive the acute stroke with important neurologic abnormalities.

Previously there had been no tests that could objectively prove that a specific treatment given after a stroke improved recovery. That capability now exists. Many diverse types of treatment are now used to help patients recover. These include various drugs and herbs; physical and occupational therapies; magnetic stimulation; constraint of the preserved limbs to encourage use of the weak limbs; and different musical, art, and speech therapies. Most patients improve naturally after stroke. Therapy and therapists have large placebo effects. Patients want to believe that the treatment that they receive helps. Now and in the future, it will be possible to test objectively whether a specific drug, treatment, or approach improves recovery, has little effect, or even impedes and delays it. We know that some drugs (e.g., haloperidol) do seriously retard recovery from stroke. Present therapies as well as new treatments and approaches will be more extensively tested in the years to come.

Genetics

During the last quarter-century, there has been a revolution in molecular biology and genetics. Genetic influences clearly have a large role in determining who will develop strokes and which type of stroke they will have. The genetics of stroke and cerebrovascular diseases is complex because the causes and risk factors for stroke are so diverse. Genes that make an individual more prone to high blood pressure, diabetes, high cholesterol, heart attacks, and other general conditions also increase the risk of stroke. A number of genetic disorders have been shown to cause abnormal bleeding and increased coagulability. Many genes are important, not just one "stroke gene." Genetic analysis of some mutations has become instrumental in the diagnosis and understanding of some specific and rare genetic and mitochondrial diseases. The ensuing years will undoubtedly witness further advances in genetics. Pinpointing the genetic causes and influences on cerebrovascular disease can help the patients' relatives and progeny as well as themselves. Genetics can also provide a window into potential future treatments.

Chapter 16

Case Summaries

Robert H., a 68-year-old retired engineer, lived with his wife. His three children were married and no longer lived at home. He had had many health problems during the past. His blood pressure was discovered to be high 20 years ago. He had been given a number of different pills but high blood pressure remained a problem that was not always well controlled. Ten years ago he had a heart attack and had to have surgery on his coronary arteries. For the past few years he has felt pain in the right calf of his leg when he walks. His doctors told him that an artery to that leg had narrowed. Similar blood pressure and heart problems had led to his father dying at age 51. His brother also had hypertension and had had several heart attacks. One sister had had a stroke.

One day at work, Robert noticed that his left hand and arm felt numb and that he could not hold objects in that hand. The weakness and numbness lasted about 15 minutes. He assumed that he had leaned on that hand. Two days later, shortly after he awakened in the morning, his left face and hand felt numb and tingly for about 5 minutes. That afternoon, a shade seemed to come over his right eye and he could not see from that eye for about a minute. These symptoms worried him and he scheduled appointments with his eye doctor and primary physician. Two days later, before he saw either doctor, when he tried to get out of bed in the morning he fell on the floor. His wife heard the fall and rushed to him. She recognized that his left limbs could not move, but Robert seemed unaware of the nature of the problem. She called an ambulance and rushed him to the emergency room of the hospital.

When he was examined at the hospital, his left face, arm, hand, and leg were weak. He could not feel touch well on the left side of the body. He could not localize touch or the places where a pin was applied to his left arm or leg. He seemed unaware that there was anything wrong with his left limbs. When shown a paragraph, he omitted the words on the left. He did not see individuals on the left side of pictures shown to him. He could not draw or copy well.

Robert's blood pressure was 135/85 and his pulse was normal (80 beats per minute [bpm]) and regular. His heart was not enlarged. He had a slight short bruit (abnormal sound) over his left carotid artery in the neck. His atherosclerotic risk factors made it very likely that he had developed atherosclerotic disease in arteries that supply the brain as well as in the coronary arteries that nourished his heart. Recall that he had had a heart attack and coronary artery surgery in the past. In Caucasian men, the arteries that most commonly develop severe atherosclerotic changes are the internal carotid arteries in the neck. The episode of transient vision loss in the right eye localizes the lesion to the right internal carotid artery before it gives off the ophthalmic artery, the artery that supplies the eye. The working impression was a severe occlusive atherosclerotic lesion affecting the right carotid artery in the neck. From the clinical information it would not be possible to tell if that artery was completely occluded or just severely narrowed. The lesion in the artery was the source of an embolus that had broken loose and blocked the right middle cerebral artery, causing a major infarct in the territory of that artery in the right cerebral hemisphere of Robert's brain.

Brain imaging showed a large infarct in the right cerebral hemisphere. Figure 9-1 is a CT scan that shows the temporal lobe portion of the infarct. An MRA (Figure 9-7a) showed an occluded right internal carotid artery in the neck and an irregular plaque in the left internal carotid artery just after its origin from the left common carotid artery. A duplex ultrasound confirmed that the right internal carotid artery was occluded. TCD showed low blood flow velocities over the right eye, indicating low pressures in the intracranial portion of the right internal carotid artery.

Robert was told to continue the aspirin treatment that had been prescribed for his coronary artery disease. We considered anticoagulants to try and prevent further embolism of the right internal carotid artery thrombus, but we decided against their use. The large infarct represented a risk of hemorrhage and worsening of his already severe neurologic deficit. Furthermore, almost the entire territory supplied by the right middle cerebral artery was already irreversibly damaged. There was little territory left to save. We increased his dose of statin to try and prevent further atherosclerotic damage to his coronary, left carotid, and other brain- and limb-supplying arteries. He was transferred to a rehabilitation hospital to enhance recovery and to readapt him to his home environment.

Claire H., a 29-year-old lawyer, began to notice intermittent pain in her left face and neck. The pain was often sharp and was sometimes accompanied by headache. She lived at home with her husband and two small children. She was very athletic and played ice hockey on a team several nights a week. Her health had been excellent. She took no medications and a recent checkup showed no health problems. One of her uncles has had lung cancer, but there was no history of heart disease or stroke in her parents, their siblings, or her three brothers, all of whom were older than her.

Three days after the onset of the neck and face pain, Claire began to hear a pulsing sound in her left ear. Later that day, her right hand and arm went weak and she could not speak well. Her husband collected her at work and drove her to the hospital.

When she was first examined at the hospital, her right arm and hand were weak and her right lower face was slightly flatter than her left face. Her speech contained some wrong words and she made errors when she read or wrote. She had difficulty understanding complex phrases and directions, and she made errors when she tried to repeat phrases spoken to her. These findings indicated an abnormality in her left cerebral hemisphere in an area surrounding the sylvian fissure.

Her blood pressure and pulse were normal and there were no abnormalities on the examination of her heart. A bruit was heard over the left carotid artery in the neck and over the left eye. Clearly she had developed an abnormality in her left carotid artery. A thrombus had formed there and embolized to her left middle cerebral artery, causing infarction. Her relatively young age and absence of risk factors made it quite unlikely that the abnormality was atherosclerotic. Sudden head and neck motions and trauma during athletics can cause tearing of arteries in the neck. The most likely explanation for her carotid artery lesion was a dissection (tear) in the carotid artery in the neck acquired during an athletic event.

CT examination showed a relatively small paracentral infarct in the left cerebral hemisphere. An MRI-DWI showed the infarct more clearly (Figure 9-2, right) A CT angiogram showed a tear within her left internal carotid artery in the pharynx before the artery entered into the skull.

Claire was treated with anticoagulants. We administered dabigatran (Pradaxa), a very effective anticoagulant that works rapidly and is given in a standard dose twice a day about 12 hours apart. After 6 weeks, her CTA was repeated, and it showed that the narrowing of the artery in the area of the tear had improved. Dabigatran was stopped and aspirin (325 mg/day) was substituted.

The weakness of the right hand and arm cleared up quickly during the first few days in the hospital. She did have some slight residual numbness of the hand, but this did not interfere with her using utensils to eat, using a pen to write, or typing on a computer keyboard. She was able to return home and resume all of her household and maternal activities. Claire's language disabilities improved dramatically during the next several months. She did have speech therapy; she still had a minor degree of difficulty with names, but she was able to return to her work as a lawyer. She walks, runs, and swims, but no longer plays hockey.

Tom M., a 61-year-old single man, became ill at work. He was a longshoreman who did heavy physical work. While straining to lift some heavy cargo, he felt dizzy and lurched to his left. He staggered and seemed "drunk" to his coworkers. Several minutes later he vomited and reported that he had developed a bad headache in the back of his head and pain in his left neck and shoulder.

In the past he had been healthy, but he admitted to drinking wine rather heavily. He did not visit doctors regularly. When checked by the company doctor 4 years previously, Tom was told that his blood pressure was "a bit high" and would need to be rechecked, but he had not followed through.

When examined at the hospital, Tom's blood pressure was 200/125. His pulse was normal (72 bpm) and regular. His heart was slightly enlarged. Examination of his retinas showed hypertensive abnormalities involving the arteries in his eyes.

Tom was alert. His voice was slurred. He could not sit without support, tending to lean to the left, and he could not stand without support. Tom's left limbs had reduced tone and were clumsy. His eye movements to the left showed nystagmus (irregular, small, rhythmic beating movements). These findings indicated an abnormality that involved the left cerebellum. His high blood pressure made it most likely that the abnormality affecting the cerebellum was a brain hemorrhage.

A CT scan confirmed that he had developed a left cerebellar hemorrhage. (Figure 9-3) The scan also revealed an old infarct near the right caudate nucleus and some white matter damage around the frontal horn of the lateral ventricles. These previously unknown areas of damage were caused by his uncontrolled hypertension and had been clinically silent.

His blood pressure was quickly brought back down to reasonable levels with antihypertension medications. He was transferred to a rehabilitation hospital, mostly for gait training, but stayed there for only 10 days. Within 2 months he was walking normally except for some pause on left turns.

Tom was urged to be very compliant with his blood pressure medications, to lose weight, and to reduce the amount of salt in his diet and the amount of alcohol that he drank. Having his primary care physician monitor his blood pressure and health were emphasized as being very important.

Elaine S. was an 82-year-old woman. Her health had always been good. She was a widow who lived a very active life and often babysat for her grandchildren. Recently she noticed episodes in which her heart beat fast and irregularly. This would last from 2 to 15 minutes and worried her, but she did not tell her doctor. One afternoon her left hand and leg suddenly went weak, and she felt tingling over the entire left side of her body, including her face. She immediately went to the hospital.

When she was examined at the hospital, doctors noted that she had atrial fibrillation. Her left atrium was not contracting normally enough to eject blood efficiently into the left ventricle. A clot had formed in her enlarged, inefficiently contracting left atrium and had embolized to a blood vessel supplying the right side of the brain, causing brain infarction. Her left arm and hand were slightly weak and she could not accurately localize touch on her hand. She was alert and had no visual abnormalities. She drew and copied drawings well. She was fully aware of the weakness in her left limbs. Her neurologic deficit was slight and improved rapidly within the first day in the hospital.

Her CT scan showed a small infarct in the paracentral portion of the right cerebral hemisphere. A CTA examination showed a sharp cutoff of her right middle cerebral artery where the embolus that originated in her heart had come to rest (see Figures 9-8b and c).

When Elaine arrived at the hospital soon after symptoms developed, a stroke code was called, and she was seen by a neurologist from the stroke team. A thrombolytic agent (tPA) was given, and within a few hours her left arm and leg had become stronger. She was later prescribed dabigatran, an anticoagulant proven to be very effective and safe in preventing further thromboembolism in patients with atrial fibrillation. She was also transferred for rehabilitation. After 3 weeks Elaine was able to return home, but she had a limp and was still a bit clumsy when she used her left hand for daily activities. She remained independent and was able to shop, cook, and clean her small apartment, sometimes with the help of one of her children or a grandchild who often slept over. She was advised not to drive a car.

Chapter 17

Planning for Your Future

Managing Your Personal Affairs

Murray Sagsveen, JD, and
Laurie Hanson, JD

We all know in theory that we should plan for unexpected family emergencies, such as the diagnosis of a chronic illness. Day-to-day matters often allow us to push this kind of planning to the bottom of our "to do" list, however. Planning for emergencies by necessity involves difficult family discussions that we might prefer to avoid. However, addressing difficult family decisions before an emergency arises is usually far easier than coping with them during an emergency.

To illustrate, consider the following example:

John visited his aging mother, Bertha, and they discussed the importance of an advance directive and a power of attorney. Bertha insisted that she did not want the family to take any unusual life-prolonging measures if something were to happen so that she could not make decisions for herself. She asked that John handle her finances if she were to become unable to do so. After this conversation, John made an appointment with his mother's attorney, and after several more discussions among the three of them, Bertha decided to sign an advance directive and a durable power of attorney. A month later, Bertha had a severe stroke that did in fact leave her unable to communicate.

If John had not started this discussion with his mother about an advance directive and power of attorney, Bertha's other children might never have learned about her end-of-life wishes. Had John and Bertha not taken the time to have an advance directive and power of attorney discussed, drafted, and signed, John would not have been able to handle even routine financial matters for his mother after her stroke.

This chapter explains the importance of planning for the future *and* provides useful information to assist you and your family with these details. You will learn ways to ensure that your affairs are managed as you want them to be managed—even if you are no longer able to communicate or make decisions yourself.

You will learn about the following:

- Informal arrangements with friends or family
- Formal arrangements with or without court involvement
  - To manage your financial affairs such as powers of attorney, trusts, and conservatorships
  - To manage your health care through health care directives, living wills, POLST, DNR/DNI/DNHs, or guardianships
- To ensure that your post-death wishes are followed regarding your property and the disposition of your body

Your Emergency Notebook

A first step in planning for emergencies is assembling and maintaining key health, financial, and other information in one place so that family members and caregivers may access the information if you are suddenly unable to communicate with them. Many organizations have developed planning guides that are free for members. But you can also create your own "emergency notebook" with a three-ring binder and a set of divider tabs. Organize your emergency notebook as follows, with tabs for separating documents into the following sections:

1. Emergency contact information
   - Spouse, partner, or significant other
   - Children
   - Siblings
   - Parents
2. Financial and legal contact information
   - Estate attorney
   - Accountant
   - Investment advisor
3. Medical information
   - Medication (recent, past, and present)
   - Contact information for both primary care and specialist physicians
   - Immunization records
   - Significant medical, dental, and eye care details (including the physicians' names and locations of medical records)
   - Allergies
   - Significant family medical history
4. Financial information
   - Bank accounts
   - Insurance policies
   - Retirement plans
   - Stocks and bonds
   - Recurring bills (for example: utilities, insurance, mortgage payments)
   - Real and personal property
   - Loans (receivable and payable)
   - Financial powers of attorney
   - Taxes (location of past tax returns and information for current tax year)
   - Safe deposit box

5. End-of-life information
   - Will and any accompanying statement concerning final arrangements for personal property
   - Advance directive
   - Organ donor information
   - Funeral and burial guidance
6. Location of key items
   - Important documents (for example: passports, military records, deeds, marriage license, Social Security numbers, titles to vehicles)
   - Photos
   - Jewelry
7. Passwords and electronic media (Passwords are vital, and given that they frequently change, don't forget to update your emergency notebook, even if by hand.)
   - Home and office computers
   - Software programs
   - Financial and medical Web sites
   - Facebook and similar pages (consider, for instance, how you want these handled after your death)

Of course, an emergency notebook is not helpful if family members cannot find or access it. When discussing the contents of your emergency notebook with family members, be sure to explain where the notebook is located.

Informal and Formal Arrangements

A second step in emergency planning is to make arrangements for events that may be anticipated or unanticipated. Depending on the circumstance, the arrangements made will be either informal or formal.

Informal Care Arrangements

Informal arrangements are temporary and can usually be made with family, friends, and neighbors. For example, if you have surgery scheduled and know that you will be unable to perform normal household chores while you are recuperating (an anticipated event), you may want to line up family members or friends to assist with your medication, grocery shopping, cooking, transportation to medical appointments, or housekeeping. You may also want them to help with financial matters, such as writing out checks, filling out tax returns, and balancing the checkbook. Such informal arrangements are very common and, in fact, make up the majority of assistance to people who are temporarily or permanently living with disabilities.

Entrusting private financial or medical information to family members or friends, however, may have unintended negative consequences. It may result in uncomfortable situations that may even have financially or medically harmful consequences. In such cases, formal arrangements are preferable. Formal arrangements may include legal safeguards regarding supervision and record-keeping, or review by an outside party to minimize the risk of exploitation by an informal caregiver. Similarly, formal arrangements may also be made to protect the caregiver, who may later be questioned regarding legitimate reimbursement for services.

Even when informal arrangements work well, the day may come when more formal arrangements are needed.

Formal Financial Management Services

When planning for the future, it is important to know what financial management services are available for your individual needs. These services are listed next, starting from the least to the most formal.

Automatic Banking and Direct Deposit

Modern banking technology, such as automatic bill payment and direct deposit, can help you with your finances. At a minimum, Social Security payments and pension income should be set up so they are directly deposited. Utilities and insurance payments should also be set up to be withdrawn automatically from your account. Doing so can prevent you from unintentionally discontinuing your health insurance or from having your electricity shut off. It is wise to have one "working" bank account, such as a checking account, into which income is deposited and from which monthly bills are paid.

To arrange for Social Security checks to be deposited directly to a bank account, you may call Social Security at 1–800–772–1213 and ask for a direct deposit form or sign up on the Social Security Direct Deposit page online at http://www.ssa.gov/deposit/. A bank can also provide you with this form. Beginning in 2013, all Social Security recipients will be required to have checks directly deposited.

Multiple-Name Bank Accounts

Adding a name to a bank account is an easy and effective way to allow a trusted relative or friend to provide informal help. By having access to the account, that person can help sign checks, pay bills, or transfer money between your accounts. That person can also have access to bank records to monitor electronic deposits, ensure that all bills are paid on time, and review monthly statements to ensure that nothing is amiss in all your accounts.

Several types of multiple-name bank accounts are available, each with different rules. Any type of account—for example, savings, checking, and certificates of deposit—may be held in more than one name. Such accounts are easy to set up just by visiting the bank. However, great care must be taken to select the appropriate type of account (as explained next) for your situation and to assure that you have selected a trustworthy person to help you.

The following types of multiple-name accounts are commonly available:

Joint Account

In a joint account, any person whose name is on the account is considered a co-owner. Each named person can make deposits and withdrawals without the other person's knowledge or consent. There are a few facts about joint accounts to keep in mind:

- The other person could withdraw all of your money without consequence or legal recourse.
- The other person's creditors could tie up the funds in the account (with a lien or attachment) until proof of your ownership of the funds is provided.
- A person's name cannot be taken off the account without that person's written approval.
- In a joint account, when one owner dies, the survivor automatically owns the account without going through probate court. This can be a benefit because the funds are immediately available to pay urgent expenses, such as funeral costs. It can also have negative consequences if the joint account holder is not your intended beneficiary.

Authorized Signer Account

An authorized signer account, or a convenience account, allows another individual to make deposits and withdrawals to your account and sign your checks. The other signer's creditors cannot tie up your account. However, as with joint accounts, there is still the risk that the other authorized signer could withdraw all your money from your account. Unlike a joint account, the account does not belong to the other authorized signer upon your death; rather, funds in this account belong to your estate—or to a named beneficiary (see later). The authority of the other signer ends with your death, so the other authorized signer will not be able to use the funds after your death.

Payable on Death Accounts and Beneficiary Designations

All checking, savings, investment, and retirement accounts allow you to designate to whom your account will be distributed at your death. Sometimes these accounts are called payable on death (POD) accounts. Both the beneficiary designation and the POD account allow for planning after your death, but these designations do not affect ownership during your life. The named beneficiary cannot make withdrawals or sign checks, so it is a useful way to bypass probate to give money to loved ones after your death.

Naming a Representative Payee

A representative payee is an individual or organization appointed by the U.S. Social Security Administration, the U.S. Office of Personnel Management, the U.S. Department of Veterans Affairs, or the U.S. Railroad Retirement Board who may be charged with receiving your income, using that income to pay your current expenses, saving for your future needs, and maintaining proper records. The Social Security Administration has a Representative Payee Program with rules and regulations to protect the beneficiary of the income. Learn more about the Representative Payee Program at http://www.socialsecurity.gov/payee. To have the authority to manage your Social Security or Supplemental Security Income benefit, a person or organization must be appointed by the Social Security Administration. A power of attorney or note from you is not good enough. Having a representative appointed provides oversight that may give you assurance that your bills and finances will be properly handled. Many professional fiduciaries and organizations serve as representative payees.

Family Caregiving Contracts

Individuals are often uncomfortable with the idea of paying family members or friends for caregiving arrangements. But changes in the Medicaid asset transfer rules over the past 15 years, as well as the reality that caregivers must sometimes give up their day jobs in order to provide the necessary level of care, have made personal care contracts an attractive option, both to make sure that the level of care is met and that children (or other relatives or friends) do not have to sacrifice their own financial well-being while providing care to their parents.

Personal care contracts must, as a general rule, be in writing and state the kind and extent of services that are necessary, within reasonable terms. Because personal services contracts involve payment for services, income paid to a family caregiver through such a contract is subject to payroll and income taxes, and caregivers should consult an accountant to ensure that the income is reported properly. Tax credits are not available for parent caregiving unless the parent is the child's legal dependent.

Durable Power of Attorney

A power of attorney is an extremely important planning tool. It allows you to appoint someone to manage all of your financial affairs if you are unable to manage them yourself. If no power of attorney exists and it is necessary to liquidate or transfer assets or enter into real estate transactions (including those of a spouse), it may be necessary to go to court to establish a conservatorship before these matters can be acted on. Establishing a conservatorship can be costly and time-consuming. Thus, everyone should have a power of attorney.

Power of Attorney Defined

A **power of attorney** is a written document in which you (as the "principal") appoint another person (the "attorney-in-fact") to handle your property or finances. The power of attorney can be effective for all purposes or for a limited purpose (for example, appointing another person to sign a deed for the sale of your home when you are unavailable). A power of attorney becomes ineffective if the principal becomes incapacitated or dies.

Durable Power of Attorney Defined

A "durable" power of attorney continues to be valid even after the principal becomes incapacitated. A durable power of attorney document must specifically state that it is "durable" and must contain specific language, such as "This power of attorney shall continue to be effective if I become incapacitated or incompetent." Generally, if the purpose of a power of attorney is to make sure that someone can manage your finances when you cannot, the power of attorney should be durable.

Care Must Be Taken in Choosing an Attorney-in-Fact

Powers of attorney are not supervised by courts, so they can be abused if the wrong person is appointed attorney-in-fact. While the attorney-in-fact is required by law to act in the best interest of the principal, it is difficult to get your money back if the person you have appointed handles your affairs unwisely. Therefore, you must choose someone you trust implicitly—a person who will *always* act in your best interests.

Creating a Power of Attorney

While forms are available free on the Internet, it is best to consult an experienced attorney to create a power of attorney. Too many times, individuals sign documents they have printed off the Internet only to discover later that the documents are invalid or do not serve their purposes. This can be a very costly error, because it may be necessary to have a court appoint a conservator to do what could have been accomplished easily with a validly executed power of attorney.

Safeguards to Protect You

You may trust a friend or family member to be your attorney-in-fact and feel confident that no safeguards are necessary. However, another option is to hire a professional fiduciary, such as a bank trust department, to ensure that your finances are handled the way you want. Either way, consider including the following safeguards in a power of attorney:

- Require that the attorney-in-fact provide an annual or monthly accounting to you, your lawyer, an independent accountant, or a trusted family member to review.
- Name two attorneys-in-fact on the document and specify that they must act jointly (for example, both attorneys-in-fact must agree and both must sign checks).
- Require your appointed attorney-in-fact to obtain a surety bond to cover the value of your property if the attorney-in-fact mishandles your funds.
- Appoint a successor in case the attorney-in-fact dies, becomes incompetent, or simply chooses not to act on your behalf.

Cancelling or Ending a Power of Attorney

A power of attorney can be canceled or revoked at any time. Each state has specific requirements for revoking a power of attorney. Your revocation should be sent to the attorney-in-fact and to any person or institution with whom the attorney-in-fact has done business on your behalf.

Remember, a power of attorney becomes invalid if the principal become incompetent or dies. However, a *durable* power of attorney continues if the principal becomes incompetent and can be revoked only by a guardian or conservator, if one has been appointed. A durable power of attorney terminates when the principal dies.

Trusts

A trust is a legal arrangement in which a person or a financial institution owns and manages assets for your benefit. The parties to a trust are the person setting up the trust (the "grantor"), the person or organization administering the trust (the "trustee"), and the person for whom the trust is established (the "beneficiary"). Often the grantor and the beneficiary are the same person.

An agreement, called a trust instrument, between the grantor and the trustee explains the trustee's authority. A trust can be created by the terms of the grantor's will (a **testamentary trust**) or during the grantor's lifetime (a **living trust**, also called an inter vivos trust). A living trust is the type of trust used to manage assets during a time of incapacity. Some trusts are court supervised, and some are not.

Trusts are not for everyone. A living trust is generally not appropriate for modest estates because the costs and disadvantages, including the time and logistics involved in administering them, outweigh the benefits. As with any planning tool, it is important to review each option for managing estates to determine the strategies that best fit your situation. In other words, one size does not fit all.

Basic Living Trust Defined

You may create a living trust during your lifetime by transferring ownership and control of your assets to the trust.

A trust can be revocable or irrevocable:

- As long as you are competent, you may change, revoke, or terminate a **revocable trust** at any time during your lifetime. A revocable trust is normally used for property management purposes. After you die, the revocable trust becomes irrevocable.

- A revocable living trust is often used as a planning tool because it allows a trustee to manage your property for your benefit during life and can also provide for distribution or ongoing management after your incapacity or death. Most commonly, in a living trust you would be both your own trustee and beneficiary. As such, your Social Security number would be used when establishing trust accounts or doing trust business. You would manage your property as if the property were in your name. A trust agreement would also include your directions should you become incompetent or die. If you have a medical condition that could result in your being unable to manage your affairs, a revocable living trust may be the right choice.
- An **irrevocable trust** cannot be changed or terminated after it has been established. It is a separate taxable entity, requiring its own tax identification number. Tax considerations may be a factor in deciding whether to make a trust revocable or irrevocable, particularly when a substantial amount of property is involved.

Care Must Be Taken in Choosing a Trustee

A trustee has as much, if not more, responsibility as an attorney-in-fact in a power of attorney. Great care must be taken in choosing your trustee. In most revocable living trusts, you would serve as trustee as long as you are able to do so. Should you become incapacitated, the "successor trustee" would take over and be responsible for management of all trust assets during your life and for distribution of those assets to the beneficiaries upon your death. Being a trustee is a huge responsibility and should not be taken lightly. While a family member or other individual could be named trustee if you are sure that person is trustworthy and capable of acting in this capacity, a fair amount of expertise is needed to handle the paperwork, tax returns, and property management tasks that may be involved. In most cities, professional trustees are available for hire, and many banking institutions have trust departments. Going over options with an attorney before naming a trustee is always wise.

Creating a Living Trust

A revocable living trust is established with the execution of a trust agreement. In this document, you would name the beneficiary (usually yourself during life), state how the property should be managed if you become disabled, and direct how the property should be distributed at your death. A living trust is much like a will in this way, and so many states require specific formalities in signing a trust to ensure that you are not being coerced or unduly influenced by someone in executing the trust. Trusts should be drawn up by an attorney familiar with drafting them.

Important Tip

Be on guard against anyone who uses high-pressure tactics to sell a living trust package. Do not deal with anyone who demands a signature right away or requires money before you have time to do additional research. Some companies only want to sell their prepackaged plans and do not assist clients in putting assets into the trust. These trusts can cause problems that will be expensive to fix.

To receive the advantages of the revocable trust, all assets must be placed in the trust or the trust must be named beneficiary.

A Revocable Trust Cannot Be Used to Avoid Paying Nursing Home Costs

A revocable trust is considered an available resource under Medicaid laws and is not a way to avoid spending savings on nursing home care. The federal and state Medicaid laws are very complicated and subject to change at any time. Do not try to use a trust without getting competent legal advice.

Trusts for Protecting Assets While Dependent on Medicaid

People living with chronic conditions may ultimately require assistance with activities of daily living (ADLs), such as bathing, transferring, ambulation, eating, toileting, and basic hygiene and grooming. This type of assistance is known as custodial care. Individuals may receive this care at home, or they may need to move to an assisted living facility or a nursing home. No matter where these services are received, they are very expensive. Medicare does not cover the cost of custodial care. Long-term care insurance policies may cover these types of costs. However, it is difficult to obtain long-term care insurance after you are diagnosed with a significant medical condition. When long-term care insurance is not available, private funds must be used to pay for the cost of care. Once private funds are depleted, many individuals turn to Medicaid to pay for these services.

Medicaid eligibility rules are complex and vary depending on (among other things) the state in which you reside, whether you are married or single, the types of services you need, and your age. As a very general rule, however, you may keep a car and your home (as long as you are living in it) and about $3000. Be aware that this amount varies from state to state. The point is, you can have only limited assets outside of your home and car. There are three types of trusts available that, if properly established and administered, allow a person with a disability to retain more than $3000 and still be eligible for Medicaid to pay for the cost of care. These three trusts are a first-party special needs trust, a third-party special needs trust, and a pooled trust. The funds in any of these three trusts may be used to purchase goods and/or services that "supplement and do not supplant" government benefits. In other words, funds in the trust may be used for goods and/or services that benefit the individual and do not replace the government benefits the individual receives. For instance, funds may be used to pay for a companion dog, nonconventional treatments, massage, companion services, a home, rent, travel, or clothing. Funds may not be used to pay for medical services covered by Medicaid. Because you can have only $3000 to be eligible for Medicaid to pay the cost of custodial care, having a special needs trust can make a significant difference in your life. Sometimes a special needs trust can make the difference between living at home or in a nursing home.

First-Party Special Needs Trust

A first-party special needs trust is a way for an individual to place his or her own money into a trust and remain eligible for Medicaid. It is called a "first-party" special needs trust because the individual's assets are used to fund the trust. Assets in a first-party special needs trust remain exempt if:

- The trust is established by a parent, grandparent, guardian, or court and is:
  - For the sole benefit of the person with the disability as certified by the Social Security Administration
  - For a person who is under the age of 65
  - Using the person's assets—this includes any assets a person may be awarded as a result of a personal injury lawsuit
- The trust is irrevocable by the beneficiary and may only be changed by the trustee if the change is necessary to comply

with a new law or decision governing first-party special needs trusts.

- The trust has a provision that at the death of the person with the disability, any remaining trust assets must be distributed first to the state as repayment for any Medicaid that has been received.

Third-Party Special Needs Trust

A third-party special needs trust is a way for a third party to give money to a person with a disability in a way that does not jeopardize the individual's eligibility for public benefits. For instance, if a parent or grandparent or best friend wants to leave money to a person with a disability, or if friends want to throw a fundraiser, a third-party special needs trust is used. Sometimes third-party trusts are set up while the grantor is alive; other times they are set up in wills. Assets or funds belonging to the person with the disability must never be placed in the trust. There is no payback to the Medicaid Agency. Rather, the grantor may state who will receive any funds remaining in trust at the beneficiary's death. Laws regarding the supplemental needs trusts vary from state to state, and a lawyer should be consulted in each state.

Pooled Trust

A pooled trust is a type of special needs trust, and for all intents and purposes it is administered like a first-party special needs trust. However, a pooled trust must be established and managed by a non-profit corporation. A separate subaccount must be maintained for each beneficiary of the trust, but, for purposes of investment and management, the trust pools the accounts. Each subaccount must be established solely for the benefit of individuals who are disabled as defined by the Social Security Administration. The subaccount may be set up by the parent, grandparent, or legal guardian of the individual, the individual him or herself, or by a court. To the extent that amounts remaining in the subaccount at the beneficiary's death are not retained by the pooled trust, the trust must pay such remaining amounts to the state in an amount equal to the total amount of Medicaid paid on behalf of the individual.

Health Care Directives

A **health care directive**, often called an advance directive, is a written document in which you appoint someone (a health care agent) to make health care decisions in the event you are unable to make them yourself.

A health care directive is now recognized as a combination of two earlier documents: the living will (a document that provides specific guidance to physicians, nurses, and caregivers about medical treatment) and a durable power of attorney for health care (a document that authorizes another person to make health care decisions when you are unable to do so).

Why Create a Health Care Directive?

You have the right to make decisions about your health care, including the right to refuse treatment, authorize treatment, and access information in your medical records. In a health care directive, you can authorize a trusted loved one, relative, or caregiver (the designated health care agent) to make necessary health care decisions according to your wishes if you are unable to do so yourself.

What Must a Health Care Directive Include?

Health care directives are governed by state law, and most state laws have several statutory requirements. Most important, a health care directive must be written by a competent person, and be dated, signed, and witnessed or notarized.

Who Can Be a Health Care Agent?

Your health care agent may be any individual 18 years of age or older who is not your health care provider or an employee of your health care provider. You should choose someone who you know well and trust to make decisions according to your wishes. It is very important to discuss your wishes in detail with a prospective health care agent before you finalize your decision. Make sure the person clearly understands your wishes *and* appreciates the responsibilities involved. You should also name a successor (backup) health care agent in case the primary health care agent is unable to act when decisions must be made.

What Is Included in the Health Care Directive?

In your health care directive, you may:

- Appoint one or more agents or alternative agents and include instructions for how decisions should be made and whether named agents must act together or may act independently
- State a preferred nursing home in the event such care is necessary
- State which medical records the health care agent can access
- State that the health care agent is the "personal representative" under the federal Health Insurance Portability and Accountability Act (HIPAA) and has the authority to access your medical records
- State whether the health care agent shall be guardian or conservator if a petition is filed
- State whether your eyes, tissues, or organs should be donated on your death
- Make a declaration regarding intrusive mental health treatment or a statement that the health care agent is authorized to give consent for such treatment

- State specific instructions if you are female and pregnant
- Give instructions regarding artificially administered nutrition or hydration
- State under what circumstances the health care directive will become effective
- State any other instructions regarding care, including how religious beliefs may affect health care delivery
- Provide instructions about being placed on a ventilator, receiving resuscitation, or other aggressive measures if there is minimal to no chance that you will recover
- State what will happen with your body at death (body identification/burial/cremation)

When Do the Health Care Agent's Responsibilities Begin?

Generally, the health care agent may make decisions for you when your physician believes you are unable to make your own decisions.

What Are the Duties of the Health Care Agent?

The health care agent is obligated to make informed, good-faith health care decisions from your point of view. The health care agent should follow your guidance in the health care directive and should seek legal help if the medical providers will not comply with his or her requests.

Can the Health Care Directive Be Cancelled or Revoked?

You may cancel or revoke the health care directive in whole or in part by:

- Destroying the document
- Executing a written and dated statement explaining what part of the health care directive you want to revoke

- Verbally expressing the intent to revoke it in the presence of witnesses
- Executing a new health care directive

Where Should the Health Care Directive Be Kept?

The health care directive must be readily available in an emergency. It should be kept with your personal papers in a safe place—such as your emergency notebook—(not in a safe deposit box unless someone else is also a signer on the box). You should give signed copies to family members, close friends, your health care agent, your backup health care agent, and your doctors so that they can include it in your medical records.

What Is the Uniform Anatomical Gift Act?

The Uniform Anatomical Gift Act allows you to donate your entire body, organs, tissues, or eyes for research or transplantation. If you do not make the gift, close relatives, a guardian, a conservator, or a health care agent may make an anatomical gift at the time of death—unless it is documented that you refused to donate organs while alive. Verification of intent to make an anatomical gift may be indicated on your driver's license.

Is a DNR/DNI/DNH the Same as a Health Care Directive?

The acronym DNR/DNI/DNH means "Do not resuscitate/do not intubate/do not hospitalize." This is a request by a patient to his or her physician to limit the scope of emergency medical care. The request is signed by the patient or the patient's proxy, and it must be ordered by a physician. It will be followed by emergency medical personnel if presented to them at the time of the emergency. You should have a health care directive as well, because the DNR/DNI/DNH is limited only to decisions regarding end of life and resuscitation or intubation and does not deal with all other myriad issues that may arise at the end of one's life.

What Is POLST and Is It the Same as a Health Care Directive?

POLST stands for Physician Orders for Life-Sustaining Treatment. It is an initiative that began in Oregon in 1991 in recognition that patient wishes for life-sustaining treatments were not being honored despite the availability of advance directives. POLST has endorsed programs in about 14 states and programs under development in many other states. It is a signed medical order that can be used by emergency medical technicians and other health care professionals during an emergency. The form is more specific than an advance directive and is signed by the patient's provider, making it a medical order. The physician must meet with the patient to go over the form and learn treatment options available for the specific disease or serious illness the patient has. Like the DNR/DNI/DNH order, POLST is not meant to take the place of an advance directive or the appointment of the agent.

Where Can I Obtain Health Care Directive Forms?

An attorney who specializes in eldercare law or has experience with health care directives can prepare a directive that is tailored to your needs.

In addition, suitable forms may be downloaded from reputable Web sites, such as the following:

- Aging with Dignity: http://www.agingwithdignity.org/five-wishes.php
- American Bar Association: http://www.abanet.org/publiced/practical/directive_whatis.html

- National Hospice and Palliative Care Organization: http://caringinfo.org/i4a/pages/index.cfm?pageid = 3289
- U.S. Living Wills Registry: http://liv-will1.uslivingwillregistry.com/forms.html
- The Departments of Health in individual states

Guardianship and Conservatorship

Guardianships and conservatorships are relationships between two people created by the court to protect people who cannot handle their own financial or personal affairs. Definitions vary from state to state. Most generally, a **guardian** is appointed for the purpose of managing the personal affairs of a person who has become incapacitated (called a ward), including making personal decisions and meeting needs for medical care, nutrition, clothing, shelter, or safety. A **conservator** is appointed for a person (called a protected person) for the purpose of managing finances, assets, and income when it has been shown that the person has impaired ability and/or judgment. If a person needs both a guardian and a conservator, one person may be appointed by the court to fill both of those roles.

A Guardianship or Conservatorship Is Required When No Plan Is in Place

A guardianship or conservatorship is necessary when a person becomes unable to handle finances or live safely without help and no previous arrangements have been made. The decision to obtain a guardianship or conservatorship should not be made lightly because it takes away the person's most basic right: to make decisions about his or her own health and welfare. The court will appoint a guardian or conservator who will handle all of the person's affairs, including perhaps where he or she will live.

The court will appoint a guardian or conservator only if a less restrictive alternative is not available for managing the personal and financial affairs of the person. It is likely that no guardianship or conservatorship will be necessary if a health care directive and a power of attorney have been put into place.

> It is likely that neither a guardianship nor conservatorship will be necessary if a health care directive and a power of attorney have been put into place.

Establishment of a Guardianship or Conservatorship

While practices may vary state by state, generally a guardianship or conservatorship is established by filing a petition with the probate court in the county where the person resides. Anyone can ask the court to appoint a guardian or conservator for a person who needs help. The potential ward or protected person must be given advance notice of the hearing and has the right to be represented by an attorney at any court proceeding, even if he or she cannot pay for the attorney. In this case, the court will order the county to pay these costs. The person requesting a guardianship or conservatorship must prove through clear and convincing evidence that such an order is necessary. This could be difficult if the proposed ward or protected person does not want a guardianship or conservatorship established.

Your Will

A **will** is a set of written instructions about how to dispose of your assets upon death. Assets are either described as probate assets or nonprobate assets. Probate assets are those assets whose ownership a court must rule on following the owner's death. Nonprobate assets are assets that will automatically transfer to another person at death such as those with joint tenancy or beneficiary designations or assets that have been placed in a trust. Probate court is the court charged with determining ownership either by administering a legal will or by state law when no legal will exists.

Not Everyone Needs a Will—But It Is a Good Idea

If property is held in such a way that it will pass through beneficiary designations or joint ownership, then a will is not technically necessary. However, a will is necessary if a person wants personal property, such as jewelry, paintings, and family heirlooms, distributed in a certain way. Tax or private family matters may exist that make it wise to use a will and probate court to administer an estate. Finally, even if there seems to be no reason for a will, having one is the best way to ensure that an individual's wishes will be followed.

SUGGESTED READING

Adams HP, del Zoppo GJ, von Kummer R. *Management of Stroke: A Practical Guide for the Prevention, Evaluation, and Treatment of Stroke*. 3rd ed. West Islip, NY, Professional Communications; 2006.

Bruenn HG. Clinical notes on the illness and death of President Franklin D Roosevelt. *Annals of Internal Medicine*. 1970;72:579–591.

Caplan LR. *Stroke. What Do I Do Now?* Oxford, UK: Oxford University Press; 2011.

Caplan LR. *Caplan's Stroke: A Clinical Approach*. 4th ed. Philadelphia: Saunders-Elsevier; 2009.

Caplan LR, van Gijn J, eds. *Stroke Syndromes*. 3rd ed. Cambridge, UK: Cambridge University Press, 2012.

Fields WS, Lemak NA. *A History of Stroke: Its Recognition and Treatment*. New York: Oxford University Press; 1989.

Friedlander WJ. About three old men: an inquiry into how cerebral atherosclerosis has altered world politics. *Stroke* 1972;3:467–473.

Goldszmidt AJ, Caplan LR. *Stroke Essentials*. 2nd ed. Sudbury, MA: Jones and Bartlett; 2010.

Gorelick PB, Alter M. *The Prevention of Stroke*. Boca Raton, FL: Parthenon; 2002.

Hennerici MG, Daffertshofer M, Caplan LR, Szabo K. *Case Studies in Stroke*. Cambridge, UK: Cambridge University Press; 2007.

Hodgins E. *Episode: Report on the Accident Inside My Skull*. New York: Atheneum; 1964.

Hutton C. *After a Stroke: 300 Tips for Making Life Easier.* New York: Demos Medical Publishing; 2005.

Hutton C, Caplan LR. *Striking Back at Stroke: A Doctor-Patient Journal.* New York: Dana Press; 2003.

Marler JR. *Stroke for Dummies.* Hoboken, NJ: Wiley; 2005

Senelick RC. *Living with Stroke: A Guide for Families.* 4th rev ed. Birmingham: HealthSouth Press; 2010.

Spence D, Barnett HJM. *Stroke Prevention, Treatment, and Rehabilitation.* New York: McGraw Hill; 2012.

Taylor JB. *My Stroke of Insight. A Brain Scientist's Personal Journey.* New York: Viking- Plume; 2009.

Williams O. *Stroke Diaries: A Guide for Survivors and Their Families.* Oxford, UK: Oxford University Press; 2010

Wityk RJ, Llinas RH. *Stroke.* Philadelphia: American College of Physicians; 2006.

GLOSSARY

Simple definitions of terms as they are used in this book. The parts of the brain are described and illustrated in Chapter 2, and specific arteries are defined in Chapter 3. See those chapters for further anatomical information.

Abulia: Lack of activity, initiative, or motivation.

Adventitia: The outer layer of an artery.

Afferent: An adjective that means directed *toward* a center, receptor, or organ (see also *efferent*).

Agraphia: The inability to write.

Alexia: The inability to read.

Amnesia: Loss of memory.

Analgesia: Lack of pain perception.

Anesthesia: Lack of the feeling of touch in the limbs or body. Also of course refers to making a person insensate by administering a drug or a local injection.

Aneurysm: An outpouching from an artery.

Angioplasty: Mechanically dilating an artery with an instrument.

Anomia: Difficulty in naming.

Anticoagulants: Substances that reduce the tendency of blood to clot.

Antiplatelet agents: Substances that reduce the tendency of blood platelets to stick together, to stick to the lining of blood vessels, and to secrete substances that induce blood clotting.

Aorta: The large artery that extends directly from the heart and travels down the trunk, giving off major branches to the head, chest, abdomen, and limbs. It is the largest and most important artery in the body.

Aortic insufficiency: Regurgitation of blood from the aorta back into the left ventricle due to an incompetent closure of the aortic valve.

Aortic stenosis: Severe narrowing of the aortic valve, potentially obstructing outflow from the left ventricle of the heart.

Aortic valve: The heart valve that separates the left ventricle of the heart from the aorta. When it opens it allows blood pumped by the heart to enter the aorta. Closure prevents reflux back into the heart.

Aphasia: A disability in the use of language involving production or comprehension.

Apoplexy: An old term for stroke.

Arachnoid: A spidery membrane that surrounds the brain and spinal cord. It is the middle of three membranes called the *meninges*. It lies outside of the pia mater and inside of the dura mater.

Arteries: Thick-walled blood vessels that bring blood from the heart to the various organs. Specific arteries that supply the brain are described in Chapter 3.

Coronary arteries: The arteries that supply the heart with blood.

Pulmonary arteries: The arteries that supply the lungs with blood.

Arteriopathy: A general term used to describe an abnormality in the arteries that supply an organ.

Arteriosclerosis/Atherosclerosis: Degenerative changes in the arteries of the body that lead to stiffening, plaque formation, and narrowing of the arteries.

Arteriovenous malformation: A vascular abnormality in which blood travels directly from arteries to veins without any intervening capillary network.

Arrhythmia: An abnormal heart rhythm: too fast (tachycardia), too slow (bradycardia), or irregular.

Asphyxia: A condition of severely deficient oxygen supply that arises from being unable to breathe normally.

Atheromatous plaque: A flat or protruding bulge in the lining of an artery caused by a degenerative process called atherosclerosis.

Atrial fibrillation: Irregular contractions of the atria of the heart, producing an irregular cardiac rhythm.

Atrium: One of two upper chambers of the heart.

Autoregulation: The intrinsic ability of the brain to deliver constant blood flow to a local region despite changes in perfusion.

Brainstem: The portion of the brain that connects the cerebral hemispheres above and the spinal cord below. It contains the nerve cells that supply the head and neck structures, and is a pathway through which fibers pass from the brain to the spinal cord, and from the limbs through the spinal cord to the brain. The portions of the brainstem are called (from below upward) **medulla oblongata, pons, midbrain,** and **thalamus.**

Capillaries: Tiny, thin-walled blood vessels that bring blood into the tissues of the body.

Cavernous angioma: A malformation within the nervous system made of capillaries and enclosed in a capsule.

Cerebellum: The portion of the brain located in the back of the head that is attached to the brainstem. It controls coordination of movements of the limbs and eyes, walking, and speech.

Cerebral palsy: An old term for nonprogressive motor abnormalities acquired by an infant or child during pregnancy or birth.

Cerebrovascular disease: Abnormalities related to the structures that supply blood to and drain blood from the brain.

Cerebrum (cerebral hemispheres): The largest portion of the brain, consisting of two halves (the left and right cerebral hemispheres).

Coagulation: The process of blood clotting.

Coagulopathy: Abnormal blood clotting.

Collateral circulation: Blood flow that is recruited to supply ischemic tissue.

Coma: Prolonged loss of consciousness.

Computed tomography (CT): A medical imaging procedure that uses computer-processed X-rays to generate cross-sectional slices of the brain.

Computed tomography angiography (CTA): A medical imaging procedure that uses computer-processed X-rays to generate pictures of the blood vessels that supply the brain.

Congenital heart disease: Heart disease present at birth.

Congestive heart failure: The inability of the heart to effectively pump out the blood delivered to it.

Core: In the context of stroke, the central part of a brain infarct; the portion that is most vulnerable to blockage of the artery that supplies it.

Deep vein thrombosis: Clot formation in a large vein in the limbs or pelvis.

Delirium: Nonproductive overactivity and agitation.

Developmental venous anomaly (DVA): Abnormal veins that develop because normal venous drainage is lacking.

Direct thrombin inhibitors: Anticoagulants that act directly on thrombin to inhibit clot formation.

Dissection: A tear within the wall of an artery.

Dolichoectasia: Elongation and tortuosity of arteries.

Doppler ultrasound: A noninvasive test used to measure blood flow by bouncing high-frequency sound waves (ultrasound) off of circulating red blood cells. Named after Christian Doppler, who first described how the frequency of sound and light waves can change relative to the motion of their source.

Dura mater: The firm, outermost layer of the meninges, the membranes that surround the brain and spinal cord.

Dural venous sinuses: Large veins located within the dura mater, outside of the brain.

Dysarthria: Difficulty pronouncing words.

Dysphagia: Difficulty swallowing.

Echocardiography: Study of the heart using ultrasound. This may be performed by examinations using chest probes (transthoracic echocardiogram) or by using an ultrasound probe in the esophagus behind the heart.

Efferent: An adjective that means directed *away from* a center, receptor, or organ (see also *afferent*).

Electrocardiogram (ECG or often **EKG):** A recording of the heart's electrical activity, showing pulse rate and heart rhythm. The recording is performed by placing small probes on the chest and body.

Electroencephalogram (EEG): A recording of the brain's electrical activity. The recording is performed by placing small probes over the scalp.

Embolism: The process of a particle, often a blood clot (thrombus), breaking off from its source (the donor site) and traveling to a site (the recipient site) distant from its origin.

Endarterectomy: Removing the inner core of a diseased artery.

Endocardium: The inner lining of the heart and heart valves.

Endocarditis: Infection of the lining of a heart valve or the heart.

Epidural hemorrhage: See *hemorrhage.*

Fabry disease: A familial genetic disease in which chemical substances are stored in the heart, kidneys, nerves, and blood vessels.

Factor Xa inhibitors: Anticoagulant agents that inhibit activation of blood coagulation factor X, an important component of blood coagulation.

Fibrinogen: A protein in the blood that is converted to fibrin, a component of blood clots and arterial plaques.

Fibromuscular dysplasia: An abnormal condition that causes thickening of arteries because of an increase in the connective tissue within the arterial walls.

Foramen: The Latin word for window.

Foramen ovale: An oval shaped hole between the right and left atria of the heart

Heart failure: See *congestive heart failure*.

Hemianopia: Difficulty seeing in one half (right or left) of the visual field.

Hemophilia: A hereditary blood condition caused by a deficiency of clotting factor VII.

Hemorrhage: Significant bleeding from a blood vessel.

> **Epidural hemorrhage:** Bleeding into the space between the dura mater and the skull.

> **Intracerebral hemorrhage:** Bleeding directly into the substance of the brain.

> **Subarachnoid hemorrhage:** Bleeding into the space between the pia mater and the arachnoid membranes around the brain.

> **Subdural hemorrhage:** Hemorrhage under the dura mater, but outside of the arachnoid.

Heparin: An anticoagulant administered by vein or under the skin.

Homocysteine: A normal protein within the blood. An increase in the level of homocysteine can predispose to strokes. Elevation can be due to hereditary factors or can develop when levels of vitamins B_{12} or folic acid are abnormally low.

Hyperlipidemia: An abnormally high level of blood lipids (fats).

Hypertension: Abnormally high blood pressure.

Hypoperfusion: An inadequate blood supply.

Infarction: Death of tissue caused by a lack of blood flow. (The dead tissue is called an *infarct*.)

Interventionalist: A term now customarily used to describe a physician who treats conditions by introducing catheters and substances through the body's blood vessels.

Intima: The inner lining of arteries.

Ischemia: Lack of blood flow.

Lumen: The space within a blood vessel through which blood travels.

Media: The middle coat of arteries; made of connective tissue and muscle.

Meninges: The membranes that coat the outside of the brain and spinal cord. They consist of three layers (from inside out): the pia mater, arachnoid, and dura mater.

Mitochondrial disorders: A group of conditions caused by dysfunction of mitochondria, the bodies within a cell that generate its energy supply.

Mitral valve: The valve that separates the left atrium from the left ventricle.

> **Mitral insufficiency:** Regurgitation of blood from the left ventricle into the left atrium because of incompetent closure of the mitral valve.

> **Mitral stenosis:** Severe narrowing of the mitral valve to potentially obstruct outflow from the left atrium of the heart into the left ventricle.

> **Mitral valve prolapse:** Displacement of an abnormally thickened mitral valve leaflet into the left atrium during contraction of the left ventricle.

Monocular visual loss: Loss of vision in one eye.

Motor: Related to movement of a body part.

Moyamoya disease: A condition of unknown cause first recognized in Japanese girls and women in which there is premature severe narrowing of the carotid arteries within the skull. The name is derived from a description of the overgrowth of small blood vessels, which look like "a puff of smoke"—*moyamoya* in Japanese.

Magnetic resonance angiography (MRA): A medical imaging technique that uses MRI to visualize the blood vessels that supply the brain.

Magnetic resonance imaging (MRI): A A medical imaging technique used to visualize internal structures of the brain and other body organs in detail. MRI makes use of the property of nuclear magnetic resonance to image atomic nuclei.

Myocardial infarction (MI): Death of heart tissue caused by a lack of blood flow; usually due to blockage of a coronary artery.

Myocardium: The muscle tissue of the heart.

Neuroprotective agents: Drugs that increase the body and brain's resistance to ischemic damage.

Neuropsychologists: Professionals who test the thinking and behavior of individuals using a battery of tests.

Ophthalmascope: An instrument used to look into the eye.

Osteoporosis: Reduced density of bone.

Patent foramen ovale: A persistence of the oval window that connects the left and right atria in utero.

Penumbra: Brain tissue around the core of an ischemic stroke that is deprived of blood but not yet infarcted.

Perfusion: Supply of tissue with blood containing oxygen and energy.

Periventricular leukomalacia: Abnormal white matter around the ventricles in the brain. A condition found mostly in premature infants.

Pia mater: The innermost membrane of the meninges.

Polycythemia: An abnormally high red blood cell content of the blood.

Pulmonary circulation: The blood supply to and from the lungs.

Pulmonary embolism: A clot that traveled usually from the limb veins to one or more of the pulmonary arteries.

Pulmonary valve: The valve between the right ventricle of the heart and the pulmonary artery.

Quadrantanopia: Difficulty seeing in the upper or lower portion of one half of the visual field, either the right or left half.

Rehabilitation: The process of restoring a patient to their previous functioning.

Reperfusion: Restoring blood flow that had been deficient.

Risk factors: Abnormalities that increase the probability that someone will develop a condition; herein, mostly risk factors for developing a stroke.

Scotoma: The perception of a hole in one's vision.

Secondary prevention: Prevention after an event; measures to prevent a second or subsequent stroke.

Sensory: Related to reception of various environmental stimuli: hearing, vision, feeling, tasting, and smelling.

Somatosensory: Sensations that relate to touch, including perception of pain and temperature and motion of a limb.

Stroke: Injury to the brain caused by an abnormality (vascular blockage or bleeding) of the vessels that supply the brain with blood.

Stupor: A state of extreme apathy and torpor with decreased alertness and responsiveness.

Subarachnoid hemorrhage: See *hemorrhage.*

Subdural hemorrhage: See *hemorrhage.*

Stent: A mechanical device for opening arteries and keeping them open.

Systemic circulation: Blood supply to the various organs of the body, except the lungs.

Systemic lupus erythematosus: An acquired autoimmune condition that affects many organ systems, including the skin, joints, heart, blood, and brain.

Telangiectasias: Small abnormal capillaries separated by brain tissue.

Thrombocytopenia: A deficiency of blood platelets.

Thrombosis: The process of formation of a blood clot.

Thrombolysis: Dissolution of a blood clot.

Tissue plasminogen activator (tPA): A substance that activates clot lysis (breakdown).

Transcranial Doppler ultrasound (TCD): An ultrasound examination performed by using probes placed in various areas outside of the head: over the eyes, and to the side and back of the head.

Transient ischemic attack (TIA): Temporary lack of blood flow causing neurologic symptoms that return to normal within a short period of time, usually within 1 hour. Some TIAs last longer, but rarely exceed a day.

Tricuspid valve: A three-part valve that separates the right atrium of the heart from the right ventricle.

Valvular heart disease: An abnormality of the various valves between the heart's chambers.

Veins: Relatively thin-walled blood vessels that bring blood from the tissues back to the heart.

Venous varices: Abnormally dilated veins.

Ventricles: Structures within the brain that contain spinal fluid. There are four brain ventricles; a lateral ventricle within each cerebral hemisphere and a third and fourth ventricle. The aqueduct of Sylvius connects the third and fourth ventricles. The term also describes the muscular chambers of the heart that pump blood into the aorta and pulmonary arteries.

Vertigo: The sensation that an individual or the room is in motion, usually spinning or turning.

Vestibular: Refers to structures within the inner ear that govern the sensation of balance.

Warfarin: An orally administered anticoagulant.

About the American Academy of Neurology

The American Academy of Neurology, an association of more than 26,000 neurologists and neuroscience professionals, is dedicated to promoting the highest quality patient-centered neurologic care. A neurologist is a doctor with specialized training in diagnosing, treating, and managing disorders of the brain and nervous system such as Parkinson's disease, brain tumors, Alzheimer's disease, stroke, migraine, multiple sclerosis, and epilepsy.

For more information about the Academy and its resources for people with neurologic disorders, visit *AAN.com*. To sign up for a free subscription to *Neurology Now®*, the Academy's magazine for patients and caregivers, visit *NeurologyNow.com*.

About the American Brain Foundation

The American Brain Foundation, the foundation of the American Academy of Neurology, funds the most crucial research to cure brain disease, such as Alzheimer's disease, stroke, Parkinson's disease, autism, and epilepsy. Brain disease affects more than 50 million people in the United States alone. In moving toward its vision to cure brain disease, the American Brain Foundation's goal is to reduce the prevalence of brain disease 50 percent by 2040. Learn more at *CureBrainDisease.org*.

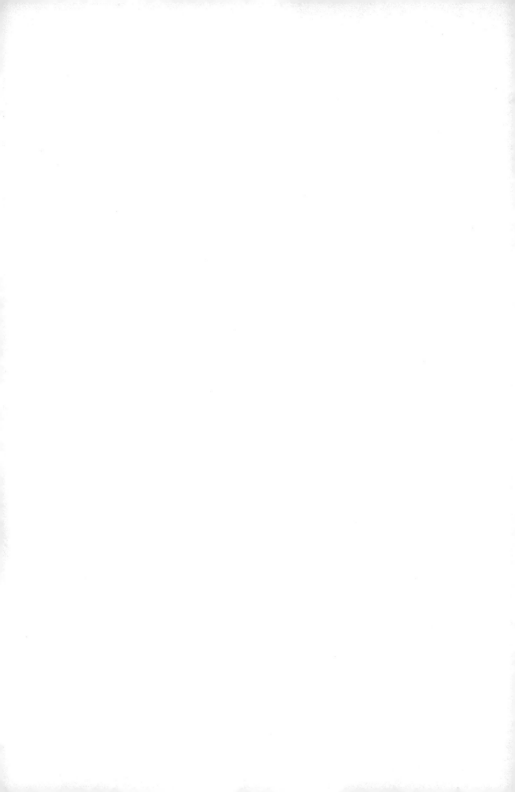

INDEX